I0493679

Future Research Needs Paper

Number 34

Chronic Venous Leg Ulcer Treatment: Future Research Needs

Identification of Future Research Needs From Comparative Effectiveness Review No. 127

Prepared for:
Agency for Healthcare Research and Quality
U.S. Department of Health and Human Services
540 Gaither Road
Rockville, MD 20850
www.ahrq.gov

Contract No. 290-2007-10061-I

Prepared by:
Johns Hopkins University Evidence-based Practice Center
Baltimore, MD

Investigators:
Gerald Lazarus, M.D.
Fran Valle, D.N.P., M.S., C.R.N.P.
Mahmoud Malas, M.D., M.H.S.
Umair Qazi, M.D., M.P.H.
Nisa Maruthur, M.D., M.H.S.
Jonathan Zenilman, M.D.
Chad Boult, M.D., M.P.H., M.B.A.
David Doggett, Ph.D.
Oluwakemi A. Fawole, M.B.C.H.B., M.P.H.
Eric B. Bass, M.D., M.P.H.

AHRQ Publication No. 13(14)-EHC034-EF
November 2013
Addendum added January 2014

Addendum to Future Research Needs Report for Chronic Venous Leg Ulcer Treatment

This report was posted for public comment from November 4, 2013 to December 2, 2013 on the Effective Health Care Web site. We received one set of thoughtful comments from the American Physical Therapy Association. The comments were related to gaps outside the scope of the original systematic review and included: the role of exercise to optimize venous pump function, optimization of general fluid balance, occupational strategies to minimize edema, inclusion of strategies for debridement and predisposing factors for venous ulcers which are located at the level of the malleoli and above. Our review involved 10,066 articles focused on the original scope of the systematic review. We agree that these issues are of importance for this very common clinical entity but our resources were limited to the original questions. Therefore no changes were made to the original report.

This report is based on research conducted by the Johns Hopkins University Evidence-based Practice Center (EPC) under contract to the Agency for Healthcare Research and Quality (AHRQ), Rockville, MD (Contract No. 290-2007-10061-I). The findings and conclusions in this document are those of the author(s), who are responsible for its contents; the findings and conclusions do not necessarily represent the views of AHRQ. Therefore, no statement in this report should be construed as an official position of AHRQ or of the U.S. Department of Health and Human Services.

The information in this report is intended to help health care researchers and funders of research make well-informed decisions in designing and funding research and thereby improve the quality of health care services. This report is not intended to be a substitute for the application of scientific judgment. Anyone who makes decisions concerning the provision of clinical care should consider this report in the same way as any medical research and in conjunction with all other pertinent information, i.e., in the context of available resources and circumstances.

This document is in the public domain and may be used and reprinted without permission except those copyrighted materials that are clearly noted in the document. Further reproduction of those copyrighted materials is prohibited without the specific permission of copyright holders.

Persons using assistive technology may not be able to fully access information in this report. For assistance contact EffectiveHealthCare@ahrq.hhs.gov.

None of the investigators have any affiliation or financial involvement that conflicts with the material presented in this report.

Suggested citation: Lazarus G, Valle F, Malas M, Qazi U, Maruthur N, Zenilman J, Boult C, Doggett D, Fawole OA, Bass EB. Chronic Venous Leg Ulcer Treatment: Future Research Needs. Future Research Needs Paper No. 34. (Prepared by Johns Hopkins University Evidence-Based Practice Center under Contract No. 290-2007-10061-I.) AHRQ Publication No. 13(14)-EHC034-EF. Rockville, MD: Agency for Healthcare Research and Quality. November 2013. Addendum added January 2014. www.effectivehealthcare.ahrq.gov/reports/final.cfm.

Preface

The Agency for Healthcare Research and Quality (AHRQ), through its Evidence-based Practice Centers (EPCs), sponsors the development of evidence reports and technology assessments to assist public- and private-sector organizations in their efforts to improve the quality of health care in the United States. The reports and assessments provide organizations with comprehensive, science-based information on common, costly medical conditions and new health care technologies and strategies. The EPCs systematically review the relevant scientific literature on topics assigned to them by AHRQ and conduct additional analyses when appropriate prior to developing their reports and assessments.

An important part of evidence reports is to not only synthesize the evidence, but also to identify the gaps in evidence that limited the ability to answer the systematic review questions. AHRQ supports EPCs to work with various stakeholders to identify and prioritize the future research that is needed by decisionmakers. This information is provided for researchers and funders of research in these Future Research Needs papers. These papers are made available for public comment and use and may be revised.

AHRQ expects that the EPC evidence reports and technology assessments will inform individual health plans, providers, and purchasers as well as the health care system as a whole by providing important information to help improve health care quality. The evidence reports undergo public comment prior to their release as a final report.

We welcome comments on this Future Research Needs document. They may be sent by mail to the Task Order Officer named below at: Agency for Healthcare Research and Quality, 540 Gaither Road, Rockville, MD 20850, or by email to epc@ahrq.hhs.gov.

Richard G. Kronick, Ph.D.
Director
Agency for Healthcare Research and Quality

Jean Slutsky, P.A., M.S.P.H.
Director, Center for Outcomes and Evidence
Agency for Healthcare Research and Quality

Stephanie Chang M.D., M.P.H.
Director, EPC Program
Center for Outcomes and Evidence
Agency for Healthcare Research and Quality

Christine Chang, M.D., M.P.H.
Task Order Officer
Center for Outcomes and Evidence
Agency for Healthcare Research and Quality

Acknowledgments

We thank the members of the stakeholder panel (listed below).

Contributors

Laura Bolton, Ph.D.
University of Medicine and Dentistry of New Jersey
New Brunswick, NJ

Anthony Disser, M.D.
Kindred Healthcare
Louisville, KY

Robert Kirsner, M.D.
University of Miami School of Medicine
Miami, FL

Peter Lawrence, M.D.
University of California, Los Angeles
Los Angeles, CA

David Margolis, M.D.
University of Pennsylvania
Philadelphia, PA

David Martin, MD
United Healthcare
Minneapolis, MN

Marcia Nusgart, R.Ph.
Patient Advocate
Alliance of Wound Care Stakeholders
Washington, DC

Robert Snyder, D.P.M, C.W.S.
Association for the Advancement of Wound Care
Quincy, MA

Charles Turkelson, Ph.D.
Center for Medical Technology Policy
Baltimore, MD

Limitations of Systematic Review

The major limitation of the systematic review was the lack of high-quality studies of sufficient size. The evidence was mostly of low or insufficient strength. Major limitations included: lack of randomized allocation; lack of masking of outcome assessors; lack of standard outcome definitions; suboptimal comparison groups; inconsistent duration of interventions; lack of statistical analyses beyond simple healing rates; lack of sample size calculations; and large losses to followup. Thus, it could not be concluded whether many of the interventions do or do not have clinical value.

Contents

Tables

Figures

Appendixes

Executive Summary

Background

Uncertainties Prompting Systematic Review

Chronic venous leg ulcers affect between 500,000 and 2 million persons annually, and over 50 percent of leg ulcers in the United States are classified as venous ulcers.[1] They are caused by elevated venous pressure, turbulent venous flow, and inadequate venous return that can be due to occlusion or reflux in the venous system.[2] The Johns Hopkins University Evidence-based Practice Center performed a systematic review[3] to determine the effectiveness and safety of advanced wound dressings, systemic antibiotics, and surgical interventions relative to either compression systems or each other among patients with chronic venous leg ulcers. We defined chronic venous leg ulcers as active, noninfected ulcers present for 6 weeks or more with evidence of pre-existing venous disease. An analytic framework was used in the systematic review to describe research gaps (Figure A). Standard therapy includes aggressive compression with debridement, which heals 50 to 60 percent of venous leg ulcers.[4] Widely used add-on interventions include wound dressings with active components ("advanced wound dressings"), local or systemic antimicrobials, and venous surgery.[5] The comparative effectiveness and safety of these advanced wound dressings, antimicrobials and surgical procedures is unclear.

Conclusions of Systematic Review

The main findings of the systematic review are summarized in Table A. The table highlights the findings for which the strength of evidence was low, moderate, or high, while also noting that the evidence was insufficient for many of the treatments of interest.

Figure A. Analytic framework for comparative effectiveness of treatments

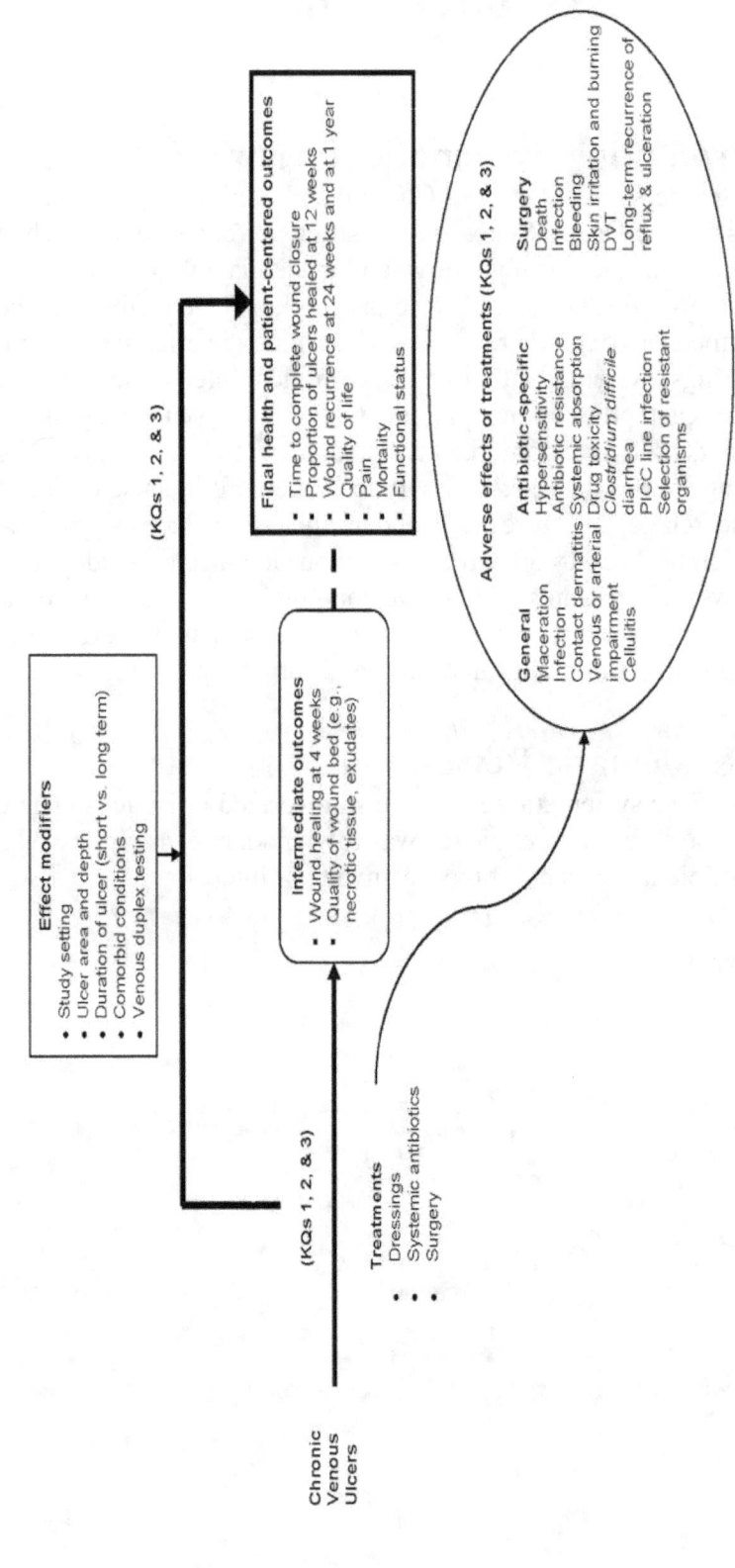

DVT=deep vein thrombosis; KQ=Key Question; PICC=peripherally inserted central catheters.

Table A. Systematic review Key Questions, findings, and strength of evidence

Key Question	Finding	Strength of Evidence*
KQ 1. For patients with chronic venous leg ulcers, what are the benefits and harms of using dressings that regulate wound moisture with or without active chemical, enzymatic, biologic, or antimicrobial components in conjunction with compression systems when compared with using solely compression systems?	Hydrocolloid dressings were not more effective than compression therapy alone in healing chronic venous ulcers. A collagen dressing produced faster wound healing than a non-collagen dressing. Cellular human skin equivalent dressings produced more rapid wound healing than compression therapy alone. Cadexomer iodine dressings produced modest improvements in wound healing rates and wound area compared with non-antimicrobial dressings. Silver dressings did not improve wound healing compared with non-silver dressings. For all other types of dressings, the evidence was insufficient to support a conclusion.	Low Low Moderate Moderate Moderate Insufficient
KQ 2a. For patients with chronic venous leg ulcers that do not have clinical signs of cellulitis that are being treated with compression systems, what are the benefits and harms of using systemic antibiotics when compared with using solely compression systems?	Only one study addressed this question, and it provided insufficient evidence to determine how the benefits and harms of systemic antibiotics compared with compression therapy alone.	Insufficient
KQ 2b. For patients with chronic venous leg ulcers that do not have clinical signs of cellulitis that are being treated with dressings that regulate wound moisture with or without active chemical, enzymatic, biologic, or antimicrobial components, what are the benefits and harms of using systemic antibiotics when compared with using dressings alone?	No studies addressed this question.	Insufficient
KQ 3a. For patients with chronic venous leg ulcers, what are the benefits and harms of surgical procedures aimed at the underlying venous abnormalities when compared with using solely compression systems?	Surgical procedures targeting superficial vein reflux produced similar rates of wound healing compared with compression therapy alone, but had lower ulcer recurrence rates at 3 years. Selected surgical procedures targeting perforator vein reflux produced similar rates of wound healing compared with compression therapy alone. One of these procedures (Conservative Hemodynamic treatment of Insufficiency of the Venous system in an Ambulatory setting (CHIVA)) had a lower ulcer recurrence rate. The evidence was insufficient regarding the benefits and harms of sclerotherapy, vein stripping, radiofrequency ablation, or endovenous laser therapy for superficial vein reflux, or surgery for deep vein disease.	Moderate Low to High Insufficient
KQ 3b. For patients with chronic venous leg ulcers, what are the comparative benefits and harms of different surgical procedures for a given type of venous reflux and obstruction?	The evidence was insufficient to answer this question due to the small number, small size, and poor quality of studies.	Insufficient

KQ=Key Question.

*Strength of evidence was defined as: High = High confidence that the evidence reflects the true effect. Further research is unlikely to change our confidence in the estimate of the effect. Moderate = Moderate confidence that the evidence reflects the true effect. Further research may change our confidence in the estimate of the effect and may change the estimate. Low = Low confidence that the evidence reflects the true effect. Further research is likely to change our confidence in the estimate of the effect and is likely to change the estimate. Insufficient = Evidence is unavailable or does not permit a conclusion.

Purpose of Future Research Needs Report

We sought to identify the evidence gaps in the systematic review, to engage a representative group of stakeholders in prioritizing the gaps, and to develop future research needs questions regarding the high-priority gaps, with some discussion of appropriate study design taking into consideration the pertinent populations, interventions, comparisons, outcome measures, timing, and setting (PICOTS).

Methods

Evidence Gap Identification

Evidence gaps were identified as components of the Key Questions in the systematic review that had low or insufficient strength of evidence.

Stakeholder Engagement for Additional Gap Identification and Prioritization

Stakeholder identification. Eight stakeholders participated in the identification and prioritization of evidence gaps. We sought input from patients/advocates, clinical experts, and payers. Stakeholders were identified from the Key Informants and Technical Expert Panel members from the systematic review, as well as new participants suggested by the review investigators.

Orienting stakeholders. The stakeholders were given a description of the project, the draft of the executive summary of the review, and a web link to the complete draft report.

Criteria for prioritization. We developed criteria for prioritizing gaps that were adapted from the Agency for Healthcare Research and Quality's (AHRQ's) Effective Health Care Topic Selection Criteria.[6]

1. **Importance.** The importance of the condition to patients (including consideration of whether that gap is of particular relevance to priority subpopulations such as pediatric patients, elderly patients, vulnerable and disparity populations)
2. **Impact.** The extent to which new research with definitive findings could potentially impact decision-making by patients, providers, or policymakers

Engagement round 1, gap list review and preliminary prioritization. In the Round 1 emailed questionnaire, each stakeholder was presented with three lists. List 1 presented the three general categories of chronic venous leg ulcer treatments: antibiotics, dressings, and surgery. The stakeholders were asked to rank these from 1 (highest) to 3 (lowest), based on the criteria described above.

List 2 broke these out into 8 specific populations, and asked the stakeholders to write in for each population the specific treatment that should be given the highest priority in future research. Stakeholders were also asked to suggest additional gaps within the scope of the systematic review, to indicate if they were aware of any ongoing studies addressing a gap, and to comment on feasibility of research to address the gap. The suggested treatments were given a priority based on how many stakeholders suggested each one. This was considered the preliminary priority ranked list of gaps.

List 3 was for study design, reporting, definitions, and other methodological issues. The stakeholders were presented with 14 items, and asked to rate each one as high, medium, or low priority. There was a comment box for each item, and the stakeholders were asked to add any additional methodological items.

Engagement round 2, final prioritization. The future research needs team incorporated the stakeholder comments and additional suggestions from engagement Round 1 into three lists for final prioritization by emailed questionnaire: (1) general treatment categories; (2) specific treatments; and (3) methodology issues. These lists included the preliminary rankings from the Round 1. Each stakeholder was asked to choose their top 5 choices in each list and prioritize them from 1 (highest) to 5 (lowest). We again asked them to base their ratings on the same criteria as in Round 1, importance and potential impact. Stakeholders were again asked to indicate whether they were aware of any ongoing studies addressing the gaps (duplication), and comment on the feasibility of research addressing the gaps.

Top-tier future research needs. A global priority ranking of the specific evidence gaps was calculated from the stakeholders' individual ratings. The global ranking was inspected by the future research needs team to determine if there was an obvious cutpoint between a top tier of questions and the remainder. If the global rankings were a continuum with no apparent cutpoint, the top half of the gaps or the top 10, whichever was fewer, were to be chosen as the top tier and considered the high-priority future research needs. After determining a preliminary top-tier cutpoint according to the score sums as described above, we reviewed and analyzed the individual stakeholder responses for the gaps on either side of the cutpoint. We then assessed which gaps had received top votes and next-to-top votes from each stakeholder, and we adjusted the cutpoint to include these number 1 and number 2 votes which indicated that at least one stakeholder felt strongly about including the gap as a high-priority need. This top tier was considered the future research needs.

Research Question Development and Research Design Considerations

To develop the future research needs (top-tier gaps) into research questions, we divided the future research needs into the clinical areas of wound dressings, antibiotics, and surgery, and members of the team with specialty experience in these areas developed the needs into research questions, taking into consideration the PICOTS framework and appropriate study design issues.[7] These were circulated to the entire group by email, and discussed and further developed in multiple meetings.

Ongoing Clinical Trials Searches

To identify ongoing clinical trials that may have addressed the future research needs, we searched the World Health Organization International Clinical Trials Registry Platform (apps.who.int/trialsearch) and clinicaltrials.gov for trials registered since the search cutoff date of the review.

Results

Evidence Gaps

Eight stakeholders returned Round 1 and 2 questionnaires. In Round 1, the stakeholders did not suggest any additional gaps within the scope of the systematic review. However, they suggested additional items they considered gaps, but that were outside the scope of the original systematic review. Because these items were not reviewed with comprehensive literature searches in the systematic review, we could not use the review to verify the extent of the gaps in evidence on these specific items. Therefore, they are not presented here in the Results section. However, the team thought it was important to determine how the stakeholders ranked these out-of-scope gaps compared with the in-scope gaps; therefore, we included them in the Round 2 questionnaire for priority ranking. The entire list, including in-scope and out-of-scope gaps is presented in Appendix C (in the full report), along with the individual stakeholder raw scores. Some of the out-of -scope gaps are discussed in the Discussion section.

In the final prioritization in Round 2, the stakeholders had a near unanimous consensus in ranking wound dressings as the top priority for future research needs in chronic venous leg ulcers (Table B). The categories of treatments in Table B to some extent have different indications. Therefore, they are not necessarily competing with each other, and comparative studies between the categories might not be appropriate. However, we wanted to get an idea of which categories contained evidence gaps that were the most important to stakeholders, so we had our stakeholder panel prioritize the general categories.

Table B. Prioritization of gaps in knowledge about general categories of treatments for clinically noninfected chronic venous leg ulcers

General Categories	Priority Rank (1 = highest priority)
1. Wound dressings	1
2. Venous surgery	2
3. Systemic antibiotics	3

Moving from the above general categories of treatments, Table C lists more specific treatment gaps, along with the final priority rank determined by the stakeholders in Round 2.

Table C. Gaps in knowledge about specific types of treatments for clinically noninfected chronic venous leg ulcers

Specific Clinical Topics	Priority Rank (1 = highest priority)
Top-Tier Topics	
1. Biological dressings containing living cells†	1
2. Collagen dressings for recalcitrant‡ ulcers†	2
3. Dressings with enzymatic debriding agents†	3
4. Laser ablation for superficial veins with reflux†	3
5. Valvular surgery for deep veins with reflux†	4
6. Ligation for incompetent perforating veins †	4
7. Sclerotherapy for superficial veins with reflux†	5
8. Topical antibiotic- or antiseptic-impregnated dressings for clinically noninfected chronic venous leg ulcers†	5
9. Radiofrequency ablation for superficial veins with reflux†	5
Other Topics	
10. Alginate fiber dressings for exudative ulcers	6
11. Hydrogels and hydrocolloid dressings for dry ulcers	7
12. Balloon angioplasty for obstructed deep veins	7

* Multiple gaps with the same priority rank had tied priority rating scores.
† Indicates top-tier topic.
‡ "Recalcitrant" denotes ulcers that have persisted for more than 6 months, despite treatment.

Future Research Needs

Taking into consideration the priorities assigned by the stakeholders to the gaps in evidence, the future research needs team developed the following list of specific research questions that need to be addressed in future clinical research.

1. Biological dressings containing living cells. For patients with chronic, clinically noninfected venous ulcers, what effect do biological dressings in conjunction with compression compared with compression alone have on time to complete wound closure, proportion of ulcers healed at 12 weeks, wound recurrence, pain, infection rates, quality of the wound bed, and quality of life?

2. Collagen dressings for recalcitrant ulcers. For patients with recalcitrant, clinically noninfected venous ulcers, what effect do collagen dressings compared with compression alone have on time to complete wound closure, proportion of ulcers healed at 12 weeks, wound recurrence, pain, infection rates, quality of the wound bed, and quality of life?

3. Dressings with enzymatic debriding agents. For patients with chronic, clinically noninfected venous ulcers, what effect does enzymatic debridement in conjunction with compression have on time to complete wound closure, proportion of ulcers healed at 12 weeks, wound recurrence, pain, infection rates, quality of the wound bed, and quality of life compared with autolytic, biological, or surgical debridement methods plus compression?

4. Laser ablation. Among patients with chronic venous leg ulcers and superficial veins with reflux, is laser ablation as effective as compression therapy alone in regards to wound healing rate and recurrence?

5. Valvular surgery. Among patients with chronic venous leg ulcers and deep veins with reflux, is valvular surgery as effective as compression therapy alone in regards to wound healing rate and recurrence?

6. Ligation. Among patients with chronic venous leg ulcers and perforating veins or tributaries with reflux, is ligation as effective as compression therapy alone in regards to wound healing rate and recurrence?

7. Sclerotherapy. Among patients with chronic venous leg ulcers and superficial veins or incompetent perforators with reflux, is sclerotherapy as effective as compression therapy alone in regards to wound healing rate and recurrence?

8. Antiseptic impregnated dressings. For patients with clinically noninfected venous ulcers, what effects do antimicrobial/antiseptic dressings compared with compression alone have on time to complete wound closure, proportion of ulcers healed at 12 weeks, wound recurrence, pain, infection rates, quality of the wound bed, and quality of life?

9. Radiofrequency ablation. Among patients with chronic venous leg ulcers and superficial veins or perforators with reflux, is radiofrequency ablation as effective as compression therapy alone in regards to wound healing rate and recurrence?

Although the stakeholders prioritized surgical research needs in the above order of interventions, we believe the most important and commonly used surgical techniques for treating venous insufficiency are: (1) radiofrequency ablation; (2) laser ablation; and (3) sclerotherapy. Ligation and valvular surgery are rarely performed. Possibly this influenced the stakeholders' interest in these types of surgery.

Ongoing Studies

We searched for ongoing studies of chronic venous leg ulcer treatments, both those still open and those closed but not yet published. We identified five studies relating to cellular and acellular biological dressings, a group of dressings nearly unanimously identified by our stakeholders as a top priority for future research needs (NCT00909870, NCT00720239, NCT00425178, NCT01199588, EudraCT#: 2007-005612-91). These trials include pilot studies as well as some that appear to be underpowered. Two of the trials are ongoing. Two additional wound dressing trials were identified. One evaluates the impact of a new proprietary absorptive dressing against wound bioburden in moderate to heavily exuding venous ulcers (NCT01319123). It is not clear if this addresses one of our future research needs. However, the study sample is non-randomized and, therefore, subject to bias. The other trial (NCT01567150) is an ongoing randomized controlled trial that evaluates wound protease levels in response to a proprietary "novel wound dressing." Wound healing (reduction in wound area and incidence of complete closure) is a secondary outcome measure. It is not clear if this addresses one of our future research needs.

Discussion

Limitations

Our eight stakeholders represented a variety of perspectives and included different types of providers that are involved in the care of chronic venous leg ulcers, but included only one surgeon. The precise priority ranking of this small stakeholder group may not be fully representative of all the providers and stakeholders interested in the care of chronic venous leg ulcers.[8] For that reason, our top tier of future research needs was large and inclusive, and we do not recommend that relative rankings within the top tier be taken as precise. It is possible that the rankings would be somewhat different if we included a larger group of stakeholders or conducted more extensive discussion with the stakeholders.

Potential Evidence Gaps Outside Scope of Systematic Review

The stakeholders suggested some items they considered gaps, but that were outside the scope of the original systematic review (Table D). Because these items were not reviewed with comprehensive literature searches in the systematic review, we could not use the review to verify the extent of the gaps in evidence on these topics.

Table D. Potential evidence gaps outside scope of systematic review

General Categories
Topical growth factors
Topical antiseptics and topical antibiotics
Specific Clinical Topics
Compression garments
Dressings with growth factors
Wound cleansing agents
Negative pressure wound therapy for edematous chronic venous leg ulcers
Arterial/venous surgery for chronic venous leg ulcers caused by mixed arterial and venous disease
Adjuvant treatments (e.g., pentoxiphylline) for all types of chronic venous leg ulcers

Gaps in Study Design and Methodology in Research

The evidence gaps were not merely due to a lack of studies, but also because of a lack of the use of study designs, research methodologies, and reporting capable of producing studies with clear results that can be compared with each other across studies and treatments. This may be as much from lack of adherence to existing standards as from lack of standards themselves. If future research needs are addressed with the same types of poor quality studies published in the past, those gaps and needs will remain.

The future research needs team and stakeholders developed a list of 16 study design/methodology items that needed to be addressed better in studies of the treatment of chronic venous leg ulcers. This list was not intended to duplicate or replace existing study design and reporting recommendations. Rather it was meant to support existing standards and to highlight items particularly lacking or specific to this field of research.

Conclusions

For this future research needs report, we divided the Key Questions in the systematic review into twelve individual components that constituted the evidence gaps within the scope of the review. We presented these evidence gaps to a group of eight stakeholders representing clinical experts, payer decision makers, and consumer advocates. In two engagements by emailed questionnaires, these stakeholders prioritized the evidence gaps on the basis of importance (severity and burden for patients and society) and potential impact on decision-making by patients, providers, or policy-makers. The top nine prioritized items, compared with the standard of compression, were chosen as future research needs:

- Biological dressings containing living cells
- Collagen dressings for recalcitrant ulcers
- Dressings with enzymatic debriding agents
- Laser ablation for superficial veins with reflux
- Valvular surgery for deep veins with reflux
- Ligation for incompetent perforating veins
- Sclerotherapy for superficial veins with reflux
- Topical antibiotic- or antiseptic-impregnated dressings for clinically noninfected chronic venous leg ulcers
- Radiofrequency ablation for superficial veins with reflux

We searched databases for ongoing but yet unpublished trials and found that none of these research needs are likely to be answered by ongoing research in the near future. Therefore, we consider all of these research questions as good prospects for those funding future research in this field, and we believe such research would substantially advance the treatment of chronic venous leg ulcers.

References

1. Margolis DJ, Bilker W, Santanna J, et al. Venous leg ulcer: incidence and prevalence in the elderly. J Am Acad Dermatol. 2002;46(3):381-6. PMID: 11862173.

2. Raju S, Neglen P. Chronic venous insufficiency and varicose veins. N Engl J Med 2009;360:2319-27. PMID: 19474429.

3 .Zenilman J, Valle F, Malas M, et al. Chronic Venous Leg Ulcers: A Comparative Effectiveness Review of Treatment Modalities. Comparative Effectiveness Review No. 127. (Prepared by Johns Hopkins Evidence-based Practice Center under Contract No. 290-2007-10061-I.) AHRQ Publication No. 13(14)-EHC121-EF. Rockville, MD: Agency for Healthcare Research and Quality. October 2013. www.effectivehealthcare.ahrq.gov/reports/final.cfm.

4. Bergan JJ, Schmid-Schonbein GW, Smith PD, et al. Chronic venous disease. N Engl J Med. 2006;355(5):488-98. PMID: 16885552.

5. Carey T, Sanders GD, Viswanathan M, et al. Framework for Considering Study Designs for Future Research Needs. Methods Future Research Needs Paper No. 8 (Prepared by the RTI–UNC Evidence-based Practice Center under Contract No. 290-2007-10056-I.) AHRQ Publication No. 12-EHC048-EF. Rockville, MD: Agency for Healthcare Research and Quality. March 2012. www.effectivehealthcare.ahrq.gov/reports/final.cfm..

6. Trikalinos TA, Dahabreh IJ, Lee J, et al. Methods Research on Future Research Needs: Defining an Optimal Format for Presenting Research Needs. Methods Future Research Needs Report No. 3. (Prepared by the Tufts Evidence-based Practice Center under Contract No. 290-2007-10057-I.) AHRQ Publication No. 11-EHC027-EF. Rockville, MD: Agency for Healthcare Research and Quality. June 2011. www.effectivehealthcare.ahrq.gov/reports/final.cfm.

Background

Context

Description of Disease

Venous leg ulcers are caused by elevated venous pressure, turbulent venous flow, and inadequate venous return that can be due to venous occlusion and/or venous reflux.[1] These ulcers affect the full thickness of the skin and are most commonly located at the ankle. Chronic venous disorders should be distinguished from other causes of skin ulcers such as arterial ischemia, pressure, diabetic neuropathy, and trauma as the management of these types of ulcers varies. Identification of the specific venous defect predisposing to a venous ulcer can often be determined with imaging and may facilitate personalized and more effective treatment of the ulcer. We defined a chronic venous leg ulcer as an active ulcer present for 6 weeks or more with evidence of earlier stages of venous disease such as varicose veins, edema, pigmentation, and venous eczema but without active infection.

Clinical Context

Venous leg ulcers affect between 500,000 and 2 million persons annually; over 50 percent of leg ulcers in the United States are classified as venous ulcers.[2] Risk factors for chronic venous disease include: age; underlying conditions associated with poor venous return (such as congestive heart failure and obesity); and conditions associated with primary destruction of the venous system (such as prior deep venous thrombosis, injection drug use, phlebitis, and venous valvular dysfunction).[1] The diagnosis of venous ulcers is made clinically on the basis of anatomic location, morphology, and characteristic skin changes. Clinical diagnosis is confirmed by functional assessment of the venous system, most commonly by venous duplex ultrasound.[3] Chronic venous leg ulcers are cared for by a variety of practitioners in different disciplines, who use a wide variety of interventions. The current standard clinical approach to therapy includes aggressive compression of the lower limb with debridement of the ulcer, which heals 50 to 60 percent of venous leg ulcers.[4] Widely used add-on interventions include wound dressings with active components (defined here as "advanced wound dressings"), local or systemic antimicrobials, and venous surgery.[5]

Current Uncertainties and Controversies in Treatment of Chronic Venous Leg Ulcers That Prompted Systematic Review

Chronic venous leg ulcers are a significant source of morbidity and mortality around the world,[5] and their prevalence will only increase as the population ages and risk factors such as obesity[6] and congestive heart failure[7] continue to rise. This public health burden necessitates identification of the best first- and second-line therapies for these ulcers. While technology and innovation have resulted in a proliferation of add-on interventions, the comparative effectiveness and safety of these advanced wound dressings, antimicrobials and surgical procedures in current use is unclear. The added benefit of these therapies to standard care with compression and debridement also remains to be established.

Systematic Review Summary

Objectives of Systematic Review

The Johns Hopkins University Evidence-based Practice Center (EPC) performed a systematic review[8] to determine the effectiveness and safety of advanced wound dressings, systemic antibiotics, and surgical interventions compared with either each other or with compression systems (as the standard of care) among patients with chronic venous leg ulcers.

The authors of the systematic review narrowed the focus to venous ulcers to minimize confounding variables. The other varieties of common cutaneous ulcers such as diabetic, atherosclerotic, neuropathic and pressure ulcers have multiple underlying confounding comorbidities. The initial goal was to examine three of the major therapeutic interventions used in ulcer care in a relatively medically uncomplicated homogeneous population. The findings are summarized in Table 1.[8]

Analytic Framework

We used an analytic framework to describe research gaps using the same format as for the systematic review (Figure 1).

Figure 1. Analytic framework for comparative effectiveness of treatments

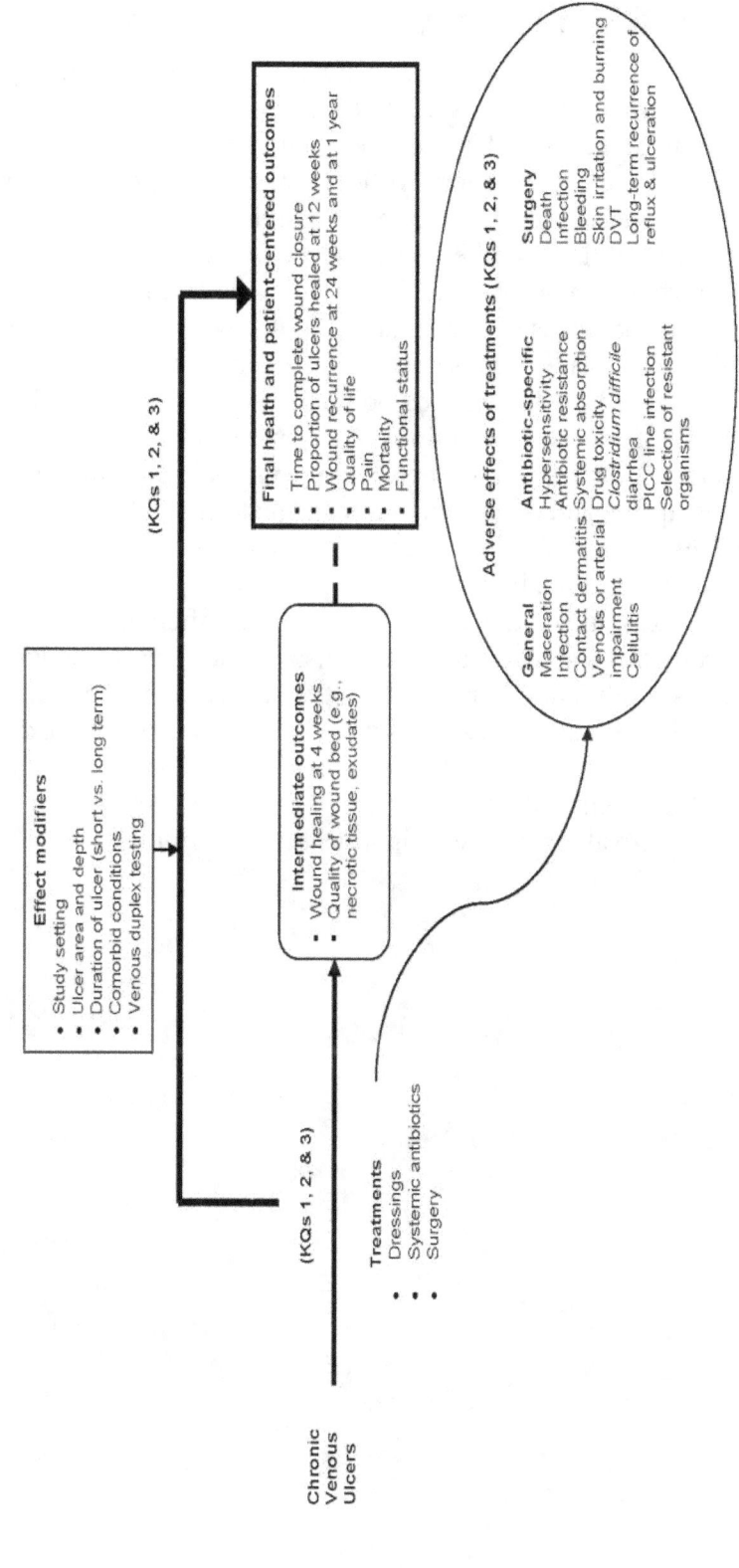

DVT=deep vein thrombosis; KQ=Key Question; PICC=peripherally inserted central catheter

Limitations of Identified Literature in Systematic Review

The systematic review[8] screened the titles and abstracts of more than 10,000 published articles, and only 66 met the criteria for inclusion in the analysis. Few well-designed randomized controlled trials (RCTs) were found that addressed the comparative effectiveness of treatments for chronic venous leg ulcers. The RCTs generally did not report on allocation concealment, and did not mask patients or outcome assessors to treatment assignment. The review was expanded to include observational studies, but these studies were largely limited to convenience populations, which, by definition, carry with them a substantial risk of bias. Overall, the studies that addressed the topic were heterogeneous and had major problems that limited our ability to make firm conclusions about the effectiveness and safety of treatments for chronic venous leg ulcers. Major limitations of the published data threatened both internal and external validity. These limitations included the lack of standard definitions of chronic venous leg ulcers, inconsistent outcome measures, suboptimal comparison groups, and inconsistent duration of interventions. Deficiencies included inadequate patient enrollment, inadequate characterization of important clinical variables, poor construction of control groups, variable lengths of study time, imprecise definitions of complete wound healing, bias and inadequate blinding, and lack of standards for measuring wound healing rates, pain, and quality of life. Studies often had large losses to followup or did not report on this. Many of the studies also did not report statistical analyses beyond simple healing rates, stratification or adjustment to account for potential confounding variables, or sample size calculations. Most studies were small and therefore had limited statistical power. Historically, case series and limited trials have been the predominant type of publications in this area of research. Furthermore, many of the interventions are classified as devices, where regulatory approval appears less rigorous than for drugs.

Table 1. Systematic review Key Questions, findings, and strength of evidence

Key Question	Finding	Strength of Evidence*
KQ 1. For patients with chronic venous leg ulcers, what are the benefits and harms of using dressings that regulate wound moisture with or without active chemical, enzymatic, biologic, or antimicrobial components in conjunction with compression systems when compared with using solely compression systems?	Hydrocolloid dressings were not more effective than compression therapy alone in healing chronic venous ulcers.	Low
	A collagen dressing produced faster wound healing than a non-collagen dressing.	Low
	Cellular human skin equivalent dressings produced more rapid wound healing than compression therapy alone.	Moderate
	Cadexomer iodine dressings produced modest improvements in wound healing rates and wound area compared with non-antimicrobial dressings.	Moderate
	Silver dressings did not improve wound healing compared with non-silver dressings.	Moderate
	For all other types of dressings, the evidence was insufficient to support a conclusion.	
KQ 2a. For patients with chronic venous leg ulcers that do not have clinical signs of cellulitis that are being treated with compression systems, what are the benefits and harms of using systemic antibiotics when compared with using solely compression systems?	Only one study addressed this question, and it provided insufficient evidence to determine how the benefits and harms of systemic antibiotics compared with compression therapy alone.	Insufficient
KQ 2b. For patients with chronic venous leg ulcers that do not have clinical signs of cellulitis that are being treated with dressings that regulate wound moisture with or without active chemical, enzymatic, biologic, or antimicrobial components, what are the benefits and harms of using systemic antibiotics when compared with using dressings alone?	No studies addressed this question.	Insufficient
KQ 3a. For patients with chronic venous leg ulcers, what are the benefits and harms of surgical procedures aimed at the underlying venous abnormalities when compared with using solely compression systems?	Surgical procedures targeting superficial vein reflux produced similar rates of wound healing compared with compression therapy alone, but had lower ulcer recurrence rates at 3 years. Selected surgical procedures targeting perforator vein reflux produced similar rates of wound healing compared with compression therapy alone. One of these procedures (Conservative Hemodynamic treatment of Insufficiency of the Venous system in an Ambulatory setting [CHIVA]) had a lower ulcer recurrence rate.	Moderate / Low to High
	The evidence was insufficient regarding the benefits and harms of sclerotherapy, vein stripping, radiofrequency ablation, or endovenous laser therapy for superficial vein reflux, or surgery for deep vein disease.	Insufficient
KQ 3b. For patients with chronic venous leg ulcers, what are the comparative benefits and harms of different surgical procedures for a given type of venous reflux and obstruction?	The evidence was insufficient to answer this question due to the small number, small size, and poor quality of studies.	Insufficient

KQ=Key Question

*Strength of evidence was defined as: High = High confidence that the evidence reflects the true effect. Further research is unlikely to change our confidence in the estimate of the effect. Moderate = Moderate confidence that the evidence reflects the true effect. Further research may change our confidence in the estimate of the effect and may change the estimate. Low = Low confidence that the evidence reflects the true effect. Further research is likely to change our confidence in the estimate of the effect and is likely to change the estimate. Insufficient = Evidence is unavailable or does not permit a conclusion, DVT=deep vein thrombosis; KQ=Key Question; PICC=peripherally inserted central catheter

Evidence Gaps

Questions in the systematic review that had low or insufficient strength of evidence are defined as evidence gaps. Based on that definition, Table 2 breaks out the individual evidence gaps determined from the results of the systematic review by the authors of this future research needs report.

Table 2. Gaps identified in systematic review

Key Question No.	Evidence Gaps	Strength of Evidence*
1a	What is the comparative effectiveness in healing by hydrocolloid dressings vs. compression?	Low
1b	What is the comparative effectiveness in healing by hydrocolloid dressings vs. other dressings?	Insufficient
1c	What is the comparative effectiveness in healing by transparent films vs. compression?	Insufficient
1d	What is the comparative effectiveness in healing by collagen dressings vs. other types of dressings?	Low
1e	What is the comparative effectiveness in healing by alginate dressings vs. compression?	Insufficient
2a	What are the benefits and harms of systemic antibiotics compared with compression?	Insufficient
2b	What are the benefits and harms of systemic antibiotics compared with advanced wound dressings?	Insufficient
3a	What are the benefits and harms of minimally invasive ligation of insufficient saphenous vein tributaries or open perforator ligation, compared with compression?	Low
3b	What are the benefits and harms of sclerotherapy, vein stripping, radiofrequency ablation, or endovenous laser therapy for superficial vein reflux, or surgery for deep vein disease, compared with compression?	Insufficient
3c	What are the relative benefits and harms of different surgical interventions?	Insufficient

*Strength of evidence was defined as: High = High confidence that the evidence reflects the true effect. Further research is unlikely to change our confidence in the estimate of the effect. Moderate = Moderate confidence that the evidence reflects the true effect. Further research may change our confidence in the estimate of the effect and may change the estimate. Low = Low confidence that the evidence reflects the true effect. Further research is likely to change our confidence in the estimate of the effect and is likely to change the estimate. Insufficient = Evidence is unavailable or does not permit a conclusion.

Comparing Tables 1 and 2, it can be seen that most of the Key Questions in the systematic review could not be answered well because of the limited quality and amount of evidence. It is promising that some of the more recent trials were of higher quality. An underlying cause of this lack of useful evidence is not lack of asking appropriate questions but rather a consequence of poor design and execution of the experimental protocols, and poor reporting. Furthermore, the team conducting the systematic review gained an appreciation of the numerous factors complicating the study of venous disease. Variations in patient characteristics might influence assignment of therapeutic interventions. Complicating variables included: ulcer size, ulcer duration, history of recurrence of lesions over time, and appearance of the ulcer base (dry versus presence of excessive moisture, hemorrhagic versus avascular, presence of fibrosis around the rim). Studies rarely reported much detail about these factors. For example, in evaluating dressings, some are engineered to absorb moisture whereas others are aimed at hydrating the base. The lack of this information made it difficult to analyze the effectiveness of the different types of dressings.

In addition, there was little concordance of experimental design across the extensive literature reviewed. Definitions of "healed and healing rates" varied substantially over duration of time. Papers often lacked power calculations for the number of patients or prospective strategies to deal with patient dropouts. Similarly, there was no agreed upon definition of durability of healing or length of followup period. Patient-reported outcomes were often uninterpretable because there were no standard metrics for assessing pain, quality of life, or adverse reactions. A substantial number of multi-center investigations were performed without evidence of standardization of observation between cooperating study sites. Evaluations of surgical interventions were often serial case series by surgeons without a control group or adequate blinding.

Venous ulcer research was often confounded by the conduct of the studies. Individual caregivers may vary in their ability to apply dressings or compression, and surgeons also have variable skill in performing procedures. To compound the complexity further, those involved in treatment were often also the evaluators of progress, which presents problems of blinding and bias.

The analysis of data varied substantially, and some studies lacked any statistical analysis. Many other studies used inadequate statistical tests. Different reporting methods prevented direct comparison of information, so meta-analysis was not possible.

Because of all these pervasive study design, methodology, and reporting issues, the future research needs team decided to list the methodology gaps observed in the systematic review (Table 3). In doing so, the PICOTS framework was used, with the addition of study design and analysis items. These two lists, the clinical evidence gaps (above) and the study design and methodology gaps (below), were the starting point for the future research needs report that follows.

Table 3. Gaps in study design and research methodology limiting conclusions of systematic review

Category	Study Design or Methodology Gap
Study Design	Estimation of sample size to achieve sufficient power; conduct and reporting of randomized allocation, allocation concealment, masking of outcome assessors, design and delivery of interventions sufficient for replication, and patient retention
Patients	Standardized characterization and reporting of patient and wound characteristics
Comparisons	Adequate comparison groups detailing level and method of compression
Outcomes	Standard definitions and measurement, including safety outcomes
Timing	Standard, sufficient duration of followup to permit evaluation of recurrence
Statistical Analyses	Appropriate statistical testing, accounting for confounding, stratification, handling of missing data and losses to followup

Methods

The aim of the future research needs project was to develop a prioritized list (or multiple lists) of research needs with considerations for potential research designs with sufficient detail for researchers and funders to use for developing research proposals or solicitations. As the resulting research is meant to improve health care decisions, stakeholders included patients/advocates, clinicians, and third-party payers.

The research needs were based on the research gaps identified in the systematic review and prioritized by the stakeholders. The methods for identifying evidence gaps and developing them into a prioritized list of research needs and feasible researchable questions involved the steps described in the immediately following subsections.

Identification of Evidence Gaps

Evidence gaps were identified in the systematic review based on the strength of evidence, applicability, and limitations of the systematic review. We started with the Key Questions in the systematic review that had low strength of evidence or insufficient evidence. A subset of seven of the systematic review authors constituted the EPC's future research needs team. The team met multiple times and circulated by email lists of potential questions to identify gaps with specific reference to study design and the PICOTS framework (lack of information or insufficient evidence for: sub-populations/whole populations; interventions, comparisons of interventions to each other; outcomes; timing of interventions or comparisons of interventions; and settings). The EPC team used this process to develop a list of research gaps to be presented to a stakeholder panel for review, as described in following subsections.

The systematic review identified pervasive issues with the design of studies that limited their interpretation. Therefore, in addition to considering clinical evidence gaps, we asked the stakeholders to consider methodologic issues in study design, conduct of studies, reporting of outcomes, and statistical analysis.

Engagement of Stakeholders, Researchers, and Funders

We recruited a group of eight stakeholders to participate in the identification and prioritization of evidence gaps. We sought input from patients/advocates, clinical experts, and payers.

Stakeholder Identification

Five stakeholders were chosen from the Key Informants and Technical Expert Panel members that previously provided advice on the systematic review. They were chosen because of their expertise and familiarity with the systematic review. In addition, four new participants were chosen to fill out the stakeholder panel. Some of these were suggested by the systematic review investigators. We also searched websites of advocacy organizations to identify patient advocates who appear to be independent of payers and manufacturers according to the voting membership requirements and funding mechanisms of their organizations. The list was summarized in a table of their individual strengths and the list was presented to the team's Task Order Officer at the Agency for Healthcare Research and Quality. Stakeholders signed a conflict of interest form declaring professional activities and financial ties relevant to the clinical area. It was made clear to them that accepting the invitation and returning the conflict of interest form constituted agreement to be identified as a stakeholder contributor to the final document. Manufacturers were not solicited to be part of the stakeholder panel, but they were informed of their ability to comment during the four week public posting period for this report.

Orienting Stakeholders

By email, we provided the stakeholders with a description of the future research needs project, and how it was related to the systematic review. We also sent them the draft of the executive summary of the systematic review. A web link to the complete draft report was provided noting that the draft was only temporarily available, and that reading the executive summary should be sufficient to meaningfully contribute to the process to identify evidence gaps and future research needs.

Stakeholder Engagement for Additional Gap Identification and Prioritization

We used an approach performed in two rounds of engagement with the stakeholders by means of emailed questionnaires.

Engagement Round 1: Gap List From Systematic Review and Preliminary Prioritization

The future research needs team's list of research gaps, derived from the systematic review as described above, was presented to the stakeholders by email for review and for suggestions of additional gaps within the scope of the systematic review. They were instructed to carry out a preliminary prioritization of the gaps, including any additional gaps they added to the list. To perform this preliminary prioritization, they were asked to use the criteria and ranking method described in the next subsection.

Criteria for Prioritization

Prior to engaging our stakeholders, we developed a draft framework consisting of criteria we considered important for prioritizing topics for future research. These draft criteria were adapted from the Agency for Healthcare Research and Quality's (AHRQ's) Effective Health Care Topic Selection Criteria[9] and included:

1. **Importance.** The importance of the condition to patients (including consideration of whether that gap is of particular relevance to priority subpopulations such as pediatric patients, elderly patients, vulnerable and disparity populations)
2. **Impact.** The extent to which new research with definitive findings could potentially impact decision-making by patients, providers, or policymakers

Other prioritization criteria were determined to be less useful or relevant for Future Research Need prioritization. **Uncertainty** is not a useful criterion, because all identified evidence gaps are uncertain by definition. **Feasibility** of research on an evidence gap is a secondary concern that is independent of the need for evidence. Evidence gaps and the need for research to close such gaps are innate to the area of interest. They are gaps and needs regardless of whether research is possible or feasible. There is value in determining the *absolute* importance and potential impact of closing each of the gaps. The feasibility of carrying out the required research to close a gap is *relative*, depending on the difficulty of the research, funding sources, availability of adequate numbers of patients, incentives for researchers, the convenience of the needed length of followup, or attractiveness of the research to researchers. A question of the highest priority may secondarily be deemed worth pursuing in spite of the difficulty and cost of the research, whereas similar difficulty and cost may render research on a lesser priority gap "unfeasible." A funding source or research group with substantial resources may consider a research question feasible, while those with limited resources may not – circumstances beyond our knowledge or control. Therefore, we did not want relative feasibility to enter into the absolute priority decisions of the stakeholders. Nevertheless, we asked the stakeholders to comment on feasibility, and we discussed it as a secondary aspect of the future research needs questions.

We did not attempt to give our two criteria quantitative values or to break these major criteria into their multiple factors for individual weighting or priority ranking and combination by a mathematical formula. That would require validation of the weights. We did not consider that practical within the scope of this project. Summing multiple factors by an arbitrary mathematical formula would give an undue appearance of objectivity, accuracy and precision. Instead we instructed the stakeholders to consider these two major criteria, *importance* and *impact*, in their priority decisions.

In the Round 1 questionnaire (Appendix A), each stakeholder was presented with three lists. List 1 presented the three general categories of chronic venous leg ulcer treatments: antibiotics, dressings, and surgery. The stakeholders were asked to rank these from 1 (highest) to 3 (lowest), based on the criteria described above.

List 2 broke these out into 8 specific populations, and asked the stakeholders to write in for each population the specific treatment that should be given the highest priority in future research. Stakeholders were also asked to suggest additional gaps within the scope of the systematic review, to indicate if they were aware of any ongoing studies addressing a gap, and to comment on the feasibility of research to address the gap. The suggested treatments were given a priority based on how many stakeholders suggested each one. This was considered the preliminary priority ranked list of gaps.

List 3 was for study design, reporting, definitions, and other methodological issues. The stakeholders were presented with 14 items, and asked to rate each one high, medium, or low priority. There was a comment box for each item, and the stakeholders were asked to add any additional methodological items.

Engagement Round 2: Final Prioritization

The future research needs team incorporated the stakeholder comments and additional suggestions from engagement Round 1 into three lists for final prioritization (Appendix B). These lists of general treatment categories, specific treatments, and methodology issues included the preliminary rankings from the previous round. Each stakeholder was presented with these lists by email and asked to choose their top 5 choices in each list and prioritize them from 1 (highest) to 5 (lowest). We again asked them to base their ratings on the same criteria as in Round 1, *importance* and *potential impact*. Stakeholders were again asked to indicate whether they were aware of any ongoing studies addressing the gaps (duplication), and to comment on the feasibility of research addressing the gaps.

Top-Tier Future Research Needs

A global priority ranking of the evidence gaps was calculated from the stakeholder individual ratings. The ratings of 1 (highest) to 5 (lowest) were inverted, so a priority rating of 1 corresponded to a point value of 5 for highest priority. Then these inverted individual stakeholder scores for each gap were summed and sorted from highest sum (highest priority) to lowest. If multiple gaps achieved the same sum, they were given the same priority rank. Appendix C shows the inverted scores, sums, and priority ranks. The global ranking was inspected by the future research needs team to determine if there was an obvious cutpoint between a top tier of questions and the remainder. If the global ranking was a continuum with no apparent cutpoint, the top half of the gaps or the top 10, whichever was fewer, were to be chosen as the top tier and considered the high-priority future research needs.

We also took into account the gaps that were prioritized highly by each stakeholder. After determining a preliminary top-tier cutpoint according to the score sums as described above, we reviewed and analyzed the individual stakeholder responses for the gaps on either side of the cutpoint. We then assessed which gaps had received top votes and next-to-top votes from each stakeholder, and we tracked how many of these number 1 and number 2 votes each gap near the cutpoint received. Using this method, we verified that the sum score cutpoint we chose reflected the high-priority items that the stakeholders sought to identify. If a stakeholder scored an item as one of the top two priorities, it was placed on the high-priority list automatically. There were 12 designated top priority gaps in the clinical evidence gaps list, and these were designated as the future research needs. However, two of the general categories and three of the specific treatment gaps which had been suggested by stakeholders in Round 1 were outside the scope of the systematic review. Since there was no systematic review to confirm the extent of these evidence gaps, we separated them out from the results, and they are discussed in the Discussion section. Likewise, the study design and methodology issues are not evidence gaps, and they are also discussed in the Discussion section.

Research Question Development and Research Design Considerations

To develop the future research needs (top-tier gaps) into research questions, we divided the future research needs into the clinical areas of wound dressings, antibiotics, and surgery, and members of the team with specialty experience in these areas took charge of the appropriate group of future research needs. They developed the needs into research questions, including PICOTS information and appropriate study design issues.[10] These were circulated to the entire group by email, and discussed and further developed in multiple meetings.

Ongoing Clinical Trial Searches

To identify ongoing clinical trials that may have addressed our future research needs, we searched the World Health Organization International Clinical Trials Registry Platform (http://apps.who.int/trialsearch) and clinicaltrials.gov for trials registered since the search cutoff date of the systematic review. Each article was reviewed by two people for inclusion, applying the same inclusion/exclusion criteria used in the systematic review. For each included trial, we abstracted the trial identification number, date of registry, the expected date of completion, the study name, status, medications compared, any published results, and determined the Future Research Need the study is likely to address (Appendixes A and B).

Analytic Framework

We used an analytic framework to describe research gaps using the same format as for the systematic review shown in the above Background section (Figure 1).

Identification of Study Design and Methodology Problems

According to the findings in the systematic review, knowledge gaps in the field of chronic venous leg ulcer treatment were not merely due to a lack of studies, but to a lack of the use of study designs, research methodologies, and reporting capable of producing a body of interpretable studies that produce clear results that can be compared across studies and treatments. Therefore, the future research needs team examined the strength of evidence findings of the systematic review and identified specific study design and methodology issues that need to be improved in future research in this field. The future research needs team presented the stakeholders in Round 1 with 14 study design/methodology items that needed improvement. The stakeholders suggested two additional items, for a total of 16 items. It did not seem appropriate to attempt to prioritize the study design/methodology items because they are all important and mutually interdependent. For presentation purposes, the study design/methodology items were organized according to the PICOTS framework, with the addition of study design and analysis categories.

Results

Evidence Gaps

Eight stakeholders returned Round 1 and 2 questionnaires. In Round 1, the stakeholders did not suggest any additional gaps within the scope of the systematic review. However, they suggested additional items they considered gaps, but that were outside the scope of the original systematic review. Because these items were not reviewed with comprehensive literature searches in the systematic review, we could not use the systematic review to verify the extent of those gaps in evidence. Therefore, they are not presented here in the Results section. However, the team thought it was important to determine how the stakeholders ranked these out-of-scope gaps compared with the in-scope gaps; therefore, we put them in the Round 2 questionnaire for priority ranking. The entire list, including in-scope and out-of-scope gaps is presented in Appendix C, along with the individual stakeholder raw scores. The out-of -scope gaps are tabled and some of them are discussed in the Discussion section.

In the final prioritization in Round 2, the stakeholders had a near unanimous consensus in ranking wound dressings as the top priority for future research needs in chronic venous leg ulcers (Table 4). The categories of treatments in Table 4 to some extent have different indications. Therefore, they are not necessarily competing with each other, and comparative studies between the categories might not be appropriate. However, we wanted to get an idea of which categories contained evidence gaps that were the most important to stakeholders, so we had our stakeholder panel prioritize the general categories.

Table 4. Prioritization of gaps in knowledge about general categories of treatment for clinically noninfected chronic venous leg ulcers

General Categories	Priority Rank (1 = highest priority)
1. Wound dressings	1
3. Venous surgery	2
5. Systemic antibiotics	3

Moving from the above general categories of treatments, Table 5 lists more specific treatment gaps, along with the final priority rank determined by the stakeholders in Round 2.

Table 5. Gaps in knowledge about specific types of treatments for clinically noninfected chronic venous leg ulcers

Specific Clinical Topics	Priority Rank* (1 = highest priority)
Top-tier Topics	
1. Biological dressings containing living cells†	1
2. Collagen dressings for recalcitrant‡ ulcers†	2
3. Dressings with enzymatic debriding agents†	3
4. Laser ablation for superficial veins with reflux†	3
5. Valvular surgery for deep veins with reflux†	4
6. Ligation for incompetent perforating veins †	4
7. Sclerotherapy for superficial veins with reflux†	5
8. Topical antibiotic- or antiseptic-impregnated dressings for clinically noninfected chronic venous leg ulcers†	5
9. Radiofrequency ablation for superficial veins with reflux†	5
Other Topics	
10. Alginate fiber dressings for exudative ulcers	6
11. Hydrogels and hydrocolloid dressings for dry ulcers	7
12. Balloon angioplasty for obstructed deep veins	7

* Multiple gaps with the same priority rank had tied priority rating scores.

† Indicates top-tier topic.

‡ "Recalcitrant" denotes ulcers that have persisted for more than 6 months, despite treatment.

Future Research Needs

Taking into consideration the priorities assigned by the stakeholders to the gaps in evidence, the future research needs team developed the following list of specific research questions that need to be addressed in future research.

1. Biological dressings containing living cells. For patients with chronic, clinically noninfected venous ulcers, what effect do biological dressings in conjunction with compression compared with compression alone have on time to complete wound closure, proportion of ulcers healed at 12 weeks, wound recurrence, pain, infection rates, quality of the wound bed, and quality of life?

- **Study Design:** A randomized controlled trial would be best to minimize bias and strengthen internal validity.
- **Population:** The target population includes patients with clinically noninfected, chronic venous ulcers of at least 6 weeks duration or more with evidence of earlier stages of venous disease such as varicose veins, edema, pigmentation, and venous eczema.
- **Interventions:** The targeted intervention includes biological advanced wound dressings (cellular, acellular). Adequate wound bed preparation such as sharp/surgical debridement must occur prior to application of these dressings to facilitate optimal outcomes. Also, standardized methods of evaluating the need for re-application need to be developed.
  - There are many classifications of biological dressings, including cellular and acellular skin substitutes. Dressings in this category tend to be expensive and their application intricate. Some of the biological dressings, autografts and cultured autologous skin substitutes for example, require either a donor site that further compromises patient comfort and risk of infection or a biopsy site to acquire adequate cells for growth.

- Xenografts are tissues derived from one species for use on another. OASIS Wound Matrix, a type of xenograft, is an acellular dermal regeneration matrix derived from porcine small intestine submucosa. It is indicated for use in the management of partial and full thickness wounds.
- Cellular dermal allografts use donor cells to create a matrix that is seeded with fibroblasts for the development of the extracellular matrix essential in wound healing. Many of these dressings are indicated for burns. Dermagraft, while studies show its benefit in the venous ulcer population, has only been approved by the Food and Drug Administration (FDA) for diabetic foot ulcers.
- Lastly, composite allografts are a bilayer skin substitute containing both a dermal and epidermal layer. Apligraf uses bovine type I collagen gel and living neonatal fibroblasts as the dermal component combined with an epidermal layer composed of neonatal keratinocytes. Apligraf has been FDA approved for use on venous ulcers that have failed conventional therapy for at least four weeks.

- **Comparison:** The comparison group should receive a compression system with at least two layers. It may also be beneficial to establish several comparison groups to evaluate the effects of single versus multiple dressing applications.

- **Outcome:** Important outcomes include wound healing rate at 4 weeks, time to complete wound closure, proportion of ulcers healed at 12 weeks, wound recurrence, pain, infection rates, quality of the wound bed, quality of life, and total number of applications.

- **Timing:** The healing rate should be assessed at 4 weeks, and 12 weeks is accepted as a standard for evaluating complete wound healing.

- **Setting:** It is essential that future trials take place in a setting with wound care clinicians who understand the evaluation, treatment, and management of chronic venous ulcers. Also, surgeons skilled in wound care, surgical debridement methods, and application of biological dressing need to be part of the research team. It is imperative that wound care providers receive appropriate education about the application of biological dressings and followup patient care. This includes adequate preparation of the wound bed by debridement, controlling for infection, and the application of multi-layer compression, and an understanding of evaluation criteria to determine the indication for repeat application.

2. Collagen dressings for recalcitrant ulcers. For patients with recalcitrant, clinically noninfected venous ulcers, what effect do collagen dressings compared with compression alone have on time to complete wound closure, proportion of ulcers healed at 12 weeks, wound recurrence, pain, infection rates, quality of the wound bed, and quality of life?

- **Study Design:** The best design would be a prospective, randomized, double-blind controlled trial. Prospective, randomized, double-blind controlled trials minimize information bias and can improve compliance and retention of trial participants allowing for a higher standard of scientific rigor.

- **Population:** In future research, ulcers need to be characterized by duration, size, and nature of the ulcer base. For example, patients with clinically noninfected, chronic venous ulcers of 6 weeks duration or more (recalcitrant ulcers) with evidence of earlier stages of venous disease such as varicose veins, edema, pigmentation, and venous eczema need to be studied separately.

- **Interventions:** The targeted intervention includes available collagen dressings. Collagen is the major protein found in the extracellular matrix, acts as a scaffold, and plays a key role in all phases of wound healing, including cellular differentiation and angiogenesis. Collagen provides the connective tissue matrix materials for fibroblast and vascular cell growth. In the recalcitrant ulcer, an increased level of inflammatory cells, metalloproteases (MMP's), can degrade the extracellular matrix and impede wound healing. Recent research theorizes that the addition of non-native collagen from a dressing to a recalcitrant wound may attract the excess MMPs allowing for growth factor stimulation and an increased production of host collagen by fibroblasts.[11]
    - The collagen within wound care products is derived from bovine, porcine, equine, or avian sources; however, the concentration and type of collagen can vary among the different dressings. Additionally, some collagen dressings can contain other additives such as alginates to mitigate exudate or antimicrobial agents to control infection. It is essential, therefore, to design trials evaluating healing rates and infection while being cognizant of the distinct differences between individual collagen dressings.
- **Comparison:** The comparison group should receive a compression system with at least two layers.
- **Outcome:** Important outcomes include time to complete wound closure, proportion of ulcers healed at 12 weeks, wound recurrence, pain, infection rates, quality of the wound bed, and quality of life.
- **Timing:** The healing rate should be assessed at 4 weeks, and 12 weeks is accepted as a standard for evaluating complete wound healing.
- **Setting:** It is essential that future trials take place in a setting with wound care clinicians who understand the evaluation, treatment, and management of chronic venous ulcers.

3. Dressings with enzymatic debriding agents. For patients with chronic, clinically noninfected venous ulcers, what effect does enzymatic debridement in conjunction with compression have on time to complete wound closure, proportion of ulcers healed at 12 weeks, wound recurrence, pain, infection rates, quality of the wound bed, and quality of life compared with autolytic, biological, or surgical debridement methods plus compression?

- **Study design:** The best design is a randomized controlled trial. It would not be possible to carry out a double blind study if comparing enzymatic debridement to autolytic, biological, or surgical debridement methods. However, RCTs minimize bias and strengthen internal validity.
- **Population:** The targeted population should include patients with clinically noninfected, chronic venous ulcers of at least 6 weeks duration or more with evidence of earlier stages of venous disease such as varicose veins, edema, pigmentation, and venous eczema. Additionally, there would need to be a standardized method of evaluating the condition of the wound bed to consistently report on the presence of necrotic tissue and to establish inclusion criteria.
- **Intervention:** The targeted intervention includes available enzymatic debriding agents. Debridement is an intervention in preparation of the wound bed since it facilitates optimal wound healing. There are several forms of debridement: autolytic, mechanical, enzymatic, biological, and sharp/surgical. Autolytic debridement uses the body's enzymes and moisture to selectively "liquefy" necrotic tissue. It is an essentially painless

process for the patient. Autolytic debridement can be achieved with occlusive or semi-occlusive dressings such as hydrocolloids, hydrogels, and transparent films. This process tends to take longer than other forms of debridement and is a viable alternative to patients who are poor surgical candidates. There is a potential risk of infection, as the wound bed is being occluded and may facilitate anaerobic bacterial growth.

- Mechanical debridement uses the concept of wet to dry saline dressings. Removal of the dry dressing causes detachment of necrotic tissue from the wound bed. However, this process is non-selective and will damage healthy, granulating tissues. It is also extremely painful to the patient. Hydrotherapy is another form of mechanical debridement that can cause maceration and damage to surrounding healthy tissue. For the most part, these methods of debridement have succumbed to the more selective and less painful types of debridement.

- Enzymatic debriders are chemical enzymes that help to dissolve or loosen the necrotic tissue from the wound bed. Collagenase digests the collagen in necrotic tissue while sparing healthy tissue and allowing for generation and proliferation of granulation tissue. In 2009, the FDA removed all enzymatic debriding products containing papain-urea (such as Accuzyme, Ethezyme, Panafil) due to significant side effects. Enzymatic debriders are prescription, topical medications that are costly to the patient. They can be used on wounds with large amounts of necrotic tissue. As with autolytic debridement, enzymatic debridement is a slow process and is an alternative for the patient who is a poor surgical candidate.

- Sharp, bedside debridement and surgical debridement are the fastest methods to debride a wound. They are highly selective and require knowledge of excisional practices. There is a higher risk of bleeding and the patient may experience excisional pain requiring analgesia. Depending on the amount and nature of surgical debridement, operating room time and general anesthesia may be required.

- **Comparison:** Comparisons could include treatment with autolytic, biological, or surgical debridement. It would be beneficial to specifically compare enzymatic debriding agents with sharp bedside /surgical debridement or biological debridement.

- **Outcome:** Important outcomes include quality of the wound bed (amount of necrotic tissue and/or presence of granulation tissue), time to complete wound closure, proportion of ulcers healed at 12 weeks, wound recurrence, pain, infection rates, complications, and quality of life.

- **Timing:** The healing rate should be assessed at 4 weeks, and 12 weeks is accepted as a standard for evaluating complete wound healing

- **Setting:** It is essential that future trials take place in a setting with wound care clinicians who understand the evaluation, treatment, and management of chronic venous ulcers. Also, surgeons skilled in wound care and surgical debridement methods need to be part of the research team.

4. Laser ablation. Among patients with chronic venous leg ulcers and superficial veins with reflux, is laser ablation as effective as compression therapy alone in regards to wound healing rate and recurrence?

- **Study design:** Most studies available on current surgical techniques are either case series or cohort studies with no comparisons. There is a critical need to perform well-designed

RCTs of adequate size that compare surgical treatments with the gold standard of compression therapy.

- **Population:** The targeted population includes chronic venous ulcer patients with incompetent superficial veins documented by duplex ultrasound performed by a well-trained sonographer or accredited vascular laboratory. As indicated by the term "chronic venous ulcer," there is usually an underlying pathophysiological problem of the affected veins. Matching the proper treatment to this underlying pathophysiology requires an accurate diagnosis using ultrasound performed by a well-trained sonographer or accredited vascular laboratory. Inadequate diagnosis and reporting of underlying pathophysiology confounds study results and interpretation.
- **Intervention:** The intervention of interest here is laser ablation of superficial veins.
- **Comparison:** The comparison group should receive multilayer compression therapy
- **Outcome:** Important outcomes include the rate of ulcer healing, and recurrence rate.
- **Timing:** Followup should continue for at least 12 months.

5. Valvular surgery. Among patients with chronic venous leg ulcer and deep veins with reflux, is valvular surgery as effective as compression therapy alone in regards to wound healing rate and recurrence?

- **Study design:** An RCT would be the best design for the same reasons as noted above for question 4S.
- **Population:** The targeted population includes chronic venous ulcer patients with incompetent deep veins documented by duplex ultrasound performed by a well-trained sonographer or accredited vascular laboratory.
- **Intervention:** The intervention of interest here is valvuloplasty, valve transplant or valve transposition.
- **Comparison:** The comparison group should receive multilayer compression therapy.
- **Outcome:** Important outcomes include the rate of ulcer healing, and recurrence rate.
- **Timing:** Followup should continue for at least 12 months.

6. Ligation. Among patients with chronic venous leg ulcers and perforating veins or tributaries with reflux, is ligation as effective as compression therapy alone in regards to wound healing rate and recurrence?

- **Study design:** An RCT would be the best design for the same reasons as noted above for questions 4S.
- **Population:** The targeted population includes chronic venous ulcer patients with incompetent perforators or incompetent tributaries documented by duplex ultrasound performed by a well-trained sonographer or accredited vascular laboratory.
- **Intervention:** The intervention of interest here is ligation of incompetent perforators or incompetent tributaries.
- **Comparison:** The comparison group should receive multilayer compression therapy.
- **Outcome:** Important outcomes include the rate of ulcer healing, and recurrence rate.
- **Timing:** Followup should continue for at least 12 months.

7. Sclerotherapy. Among patients with chronic venous leg ulcers and superficial veins or incompetent perforators with reflux, is sclerotherapy as effective as compression therapy alone in regards to wound healing rate and recurrence?

- **Study design:** An RCT would be the best design for the same reasons as noted above.
- **Population:** The targeted population includes chronic venous ulcer patients with incompetent superficial veins or incompetent perforators documented by duplex ultrasound performed by a well-trained sonographer or accredited vascular laboratory.
- **Intervention:** The intervention of interest is sclerotherapy of incompetent superficial veins or incompetent perforators.
- **Comparison:** The comparison group should receive multilayer compression therapy.
- **Outcome:** Important outcomes include the rate of ulcer healing, and recurrence rate.
- **Timing:** Followup should continue for at least 12 months.

8. Antiseptic impregnated dressings. For patients with clinically noninfected venous ulcers, what effect do antimicrobial/antiseptic dressings compared with compression alone have on time to complete wound closure, proportion of ulcers healed at 12 weeks, wound recurrence, pain, infection rates, quality of the wound bed, and quality of life?

- **Study Design:** Studies of antimicrobial/antiseptic impregnated dressing included in the systematic review were RCTs; however, most of them did not provide a double blinded design. Prospective, randomized, double-blind controlled trials minimize information bias and can improve compliance and retention of trial participants allowing for a higher standard of scientific rigor.
- **Population:** The targeted population includes patients with clinically noninfected, chronic venous ulcers of at least 6 weeks duration or more with evidence of earlier stages of venous disease such as varicose veins, edema, pigmentation, and venous eczema.
- **Intervention:** The intervention of interest includes antimicrobial and antiseptic impregnated dressings with agents such as cadexomer iodine, gentian violet, Manuka honey, silver, sodium chloride, polyhexamethylene biguanide, and others. Some of the previous trials experienced high dropout rates among participants, so it will be important to monitor adherence to the assigned treatment.
  - Advanced wound dressings vary in their structure and function and are prescribed to meet the needs of the wound: highly exuding to desiccated. Therefore, it will be necessary to have consistent methods of evaluating and reporting wound bed characteristics as well as controlling for the vehicle dressing in which the antiseptic is impregnated. Operational definitions of clinical infection versus colonization need to be clearly elucidated. Some dressings impregnated with antiseptics may require more frequent dressing changes, not allowing compression wraps to remain in place for 7 days. Therefore, when conducting trials on antiseptic impregnated dressings, researchers may need to standardize methods of applying adequate compression while allowing for more frequent dressing changes.
- **Comparison:** The comparison group should receive a compression system of at least two layers.
- **Outcome measures:** Important outcomes include time to complete wound closure, proportion of ulcers healed at 12 weeks, wound recurrence, pain, infection rates, quality of the wound bed, and quality of life. Wound pain can be an indication of clinical

infection. Therefore, it is necessary to develop validated and standardized scales for evaluating wound pain as well as quality of life. The development of specific and consistent methods for evaluating healing rates and quality of the wound bed will allow for synthesis of data across studies.

- **Timing:** Twelve weeks is accepted as a standard for evaluating wound healing. It is essential to standardize the timing of wound pain evaluations: prior to dressing changes, during dressing changes, between dressing changes, and so forth.
- **Setting:** It is essential that future trials take place in a setting with wound care clinicians who understand the evaluation, treatment, and management of chronic venous ulcers.

9. Radiofrequency ablation. Among patients with chronic venous leg ulcers and superficial veins or perforators with reflux, is radiofrequency ablation as effective as compression therapy alone in regards to wound healing rate and recurrence?

- **Study design:** An RCT would be the best design for the same reasons given under question 4S.
- **Population:** The targeted population includes chronic venous ulcer patients with incompetent superficial veins or incompetent perforators documented by duplex ultrasound performed by a well-trained sonographer or accredited vascular laboratory.
- **Intervention:** The intervention of interest here is radiofrequency ablation of incompetent superficial veins or incompetent perforators.
- **Comparison:** The comparison group should receive multilayer compression therapy.
- **Outcome:** Important outcomes include the rate of ulcer healing, and recurrence rate.
- **Time:** Followup should continue for at least 12 months.

Although the stakeholders prioritized surgical future research needs in the above order of interventions, we believe the most important and commonly used surgical techniques for treating venous insufficiency are: (1) radiofrequency ablation; (2) laser ablation; and (3) sclerotherapy. Ligation and valvular surgery are rarely performed. Possibly this influenced the stakeholders' interest in these types of surgery.

Ongoing Studies

We searched for ongoing studies of chronic venous leg ulcer treatments, both those still open and those closed but not yet published (see Appendix D). We identified five studies (Appendix E) relating to cellular and acellular biological dressings, a group of dressings nearly unanimously identified by our stakeholders as a top priority for future research needs (NCT00909870, NCT00720239, NCT00425178, NCT01199588, EudraCT#: 2007-005612-91). These trials include pilot studies as well as some that appear to be underpowered. Two of the trials are ongoing. Two additional wound dressing trials were identified. One evaluates the impact of a new proprietary absorptive dressing against wound bioburden in moderate to heavily exuding venous ulcers (NCT01319123). It is not clear if this addresses one of our future research needs. However, the study sample is non-randomized and, therefore, subject to bias. The other trial (NCT01567150) is an ongoing randomized controlled trial that evaluates wound protease levels in response to a proprietary "novel wound dressing." Wound healing (reduction in wound area and incidence of complete closure) is a secondary outcome measure. It is not clear if this addresses one of our future research needs.

Discussion

Limitations

Our approach to identifying and prioritizing future research needs has some limitations. Although we attempted to engage stakeholders with a variety of backgrounds, most were clinicians with experience in the non-surgical management of chronic venous leg ulcers, and only one was a surgeon. That composition more or less reflected the composition of the providers who care for patients with chronic venous leg ulcers. Even if the composition of the stakeholder panel reflected the composition of providers in the field, it is not clear that such a "majority rules" approach would identify and prioritize the gaps in the most useful way. Others have suggested that the precise priority ranking of small, informally composed stakeholder groups may have limited validity.[12] Another similarly composed group might have provided somewhat different gap identifications and rankings. For that reason, our top tier of future research needs was large and inclusive, and we do not recommend that relative rankings within the top tier be taken as precise.

It also is possible that the priority ratings would have been different if we had used a more intensive approach to engaging the stakeholders, such as in-person meetings or a series of teleconferences with stakeholders. Asking the stakeholders to read the Executive Summary of the systematic review might not have been as effective as an oral presentation and discussion of the systematic review. However, the approach we used was effective in engaging a diverse group of stakeholders in a short interval of time so that the future research needs report could be finished soon after completion of the systematic review.

The future research needs selected and presented in the Results section were constrained by the scope of the systematic review and the specific questions we asked the stakeholders to answer. Other related gaps and needs exist, as indicated by the comments that stakeholders made in the blank comment boxes we included with each item in the questionnaires. In the following section, we comment on some of those suggestions.

Potential Evidence Gaps Outside Scope of Systematic Review

The stakeholders suggested some items they considered gaps, but that were outside the scope of the original systematic review. Because these items were not reviewed with comprehensive literature searches in the systematic review, we could not use the review to determine the extent of these potential gaps in evidence. These out-of-scope potential gaps are listed in Table 6 and some of them are discussed below.

Table 6. Potential evidence gaps outside scope of systematic review

General Categories
Topical growth factors
Topical antiseptics and topical antibiotics
Specific Clinical Topics
Compression garments
Dressings with growth factors
Wound cleansing agents
Negative pressure wound therapy for edematous chronic venous leg ulcers
Arterial/venous surgery for chronic venous leg ulcers caused by mixed arterial and venous disease
Adjuvant treatments (e.g., pentoxiphylline) for all types of chronic venous leg ulcers

Compression Garments

For patients with chronic, clinically noninfected venous ulcers, what is the most efficacious level of compression as measured by the effects on time to complete wound closure, proportion of ulcers healed at 12 weeks, pain, quality of the wound bed, and quality of life?

A recent Cochrane review[13] evaluated 39 randomized control trials and confirmed compression as effective and the standard of care for chronic venous leg ulcers. Therefore, our systematic review did not duplicate this with formal comparisons of various compression treatments among themselves, but rather accepted compression as the standard for comparing all other treatments.

The Cochrane review found multi-layer compression systems (at least two layers) to be more effective in healing venous ulcers than single compression systems, and four layers of compression were considered most effective. Elastic bandages were superior to inelastic bandages. There is more to be done in deciding exactly how much pressure is best and in establishing how to quantify and report the actual amount of pressure being applied. Direct measurement of sub-bandage pressures over the medial gaiter aspect of the leg while lying supine will diminish the effect of inter-operator variability in the amount of compression applied.

Operator skill and experience in the application of compression systems can significantly affect wound healing outcomes and patient morbidity. Wound care providers must be aware of clinical indications and contraindications related to compression therapy when choosing a compression system. An additional compression therapy to consider is intermittent pneumatic compression for the non-healing venous ulcer.

Prospective, randomized controlled trials evaluating the effects of compression on venous ulcers must control for the types of sub-bandage dressings used on the ulcer, infection, and comorbidities such as arterial disease, diabetes mellitus, and heart failure to name a few.

Dressings With Growth Factors

For patients with chronic, clinically noninfected venous ulcers, what effect do growth factors in conjunction with compression have on time to complete wound closure, proportion of ulcers healed at 12 weeks, wound recurrence, pain, infection rates, quality of the wound bed, and quality of life compared with compression alone?

Growth factors play a significant role in all phases of wound healing by mediating processes such as inflammation, angiogenesis, extracellular matrix formation and degradation, granulation tissue formation and remodeling, epithelial cell migration and proliferation, and scar formation. The proteases found in chronic wound exudate create a hostile environment to the effectiveness of growth factors and inhibit the healing process.

Currently, Becaplermin is the only FDA approved topical growth factor wound treatment available in the United States. Becaplermin is approved for use on diabetic foot ulcers and full thickness pressure ulcers only. While the evidence related to growth factors was not appraised by the systematic review, the majority of stakeholders ranked them within their top two priorities for future research.

Wound Cleansing Agents

For patients with chronic, clinically noninfected venous ulcers, what effect does tap water or normal saline used as wound cleansing agents in conjunction with compression have on time to complete wound closure, proportion of ulcers healed at 12 weeks, wound recurrence, pain, infection rates, quality of the wound bed, and quality of life as compared with topical disinfectants or antiseptic wound cleansing agents plus compression?

Wound cleansing agents can range from tap water, to normal saline, to topical disinfectants and antiseptics. A Cochrane review[14] compared the use of tap water with other agents for cleansing wounds and found no evidence that tap water increased infection rates. However, there is a plethora of wound cleaning agents available and there is an obvious gap in the literature related to these agents. In a trial evaluating wound cleansing agents, wound dressings should be limited to dressings without antimicrobial properties.

Topical Antibiotic or Antiseptic-Impregnated Dressings

For patients with chronic, clinically noninfected venous ulcers, what effects do topical antiseptic dressings in conjunction with compression have on time to complete wound closure, proportion of ulcers healed at 12 weeks, wound recurrence, pain, infection rates, quality of the wound bed, and quality of life compared with antiseptic-impregnated dressings plus compression?

Stakeholders identified topical antibiotics as a priority Future Research Need, but evidence concerning the effectiveness of topical antibiotics was outside the scope of the review, so some research in this area may be completed or under way, but not reflected in this report. Antiseptic-impregnated dressings include agents such as cadexomer iodine, gentian violet, honey, sodium chloride, polyhexamethylene biguanide, and others. Of those evaluated in randomized trials, only cadexomer iodine showed a modest benefit in healing rates in a Cochrane report[9]. A focus for future research concerning antiseptic dressings is to control for the vehicle dressing in which the antiseptic is impregnated, as well as for the characteristics of the wound bed.

Current Minimally Invasive Endovenous Ablation Surgical Techniques And Sclerotherapy Compared With Historical And More Invasive Surgical Treatments

The only comparative evidence between surgical treatments is historical studies on invasive procedures that are no longer in common practice (superficial vein stripping, ligation, and subfascial endoscopic perforator surgery). The systematic review found historical evidence that the durability of remission was increased by these historical surgical procedures. These older invasive treatments are now mostly replaced by minimally invasive endovenous ablation techniques (radiofrequency and laser ablation) and sclerotherapy. These currently used minimally invasive techniques need to be evaluated to determine whether they produce similar improvements in durability compared with the historical surgical treatments. However, it is impractical to resurrect the old more invasive techniques, and that would potentially violate the equipoise required for ethical research. The only option may be the weaker alternative of the statistical technique of network meta-analysis, whereby treatment A (e.g., current surgical techniques) and treatment B (e.g., historical surgical techniques), which have both been compared with control treatment C (e.g., compression), but in different studies, are indirectly compared statistically through their common comparison to treatment C. This is a technique of unclear reliability, because it is difficult to know if the control treatment C was done with similar effectiveness in the different studies, particularly when they were carried out in different eras.

Comparison of Combinations of Simultaneous and Sequential Treatments

Our stakeholders assigned high priority to future double-blind studies comparing combinations of simultaneous treatments and sequential treatments for chronic venous leg ulcers. This is especially pertinent to surgical interventions, which frequently occur in combinations and series.

Low-Priority Evidence Gaps

Systemic Antibiotics

Determining the appropriate use of systemic antibiotics ranked last in the list of general categories of knowledge gaps, and so it was not included as a high-priority Future Research Need in the Results section. However, we mention here some salient points regarding systemic antibiotics. The systematic review stakeholders and experts largely agreed that evidence supports use of systemic antimicrobials only in wounds with clinical evidence of infection. Therefore, the systematic review only included noninfected wounds in the Key Question on systemic antibiotics. Nevertheless, they believed that antibiotics are widely and inappropriately used in wounds without clinical infection. The systematic review identified only two RCTs of antibiotics used in chronic venous leg ulcers. Both studies were more than 20 years old, had small sample sizes, and found no benefit for systemic antibiotics. The trials had inconsistent definitions of infected wounds. Infection was often confused with colonization, and the inflammation due to edema and the underlying disease was often confused with infection. These issues need to be accounted for in designing and implementing future RCTs.

Gaps in Study Design and Methodology in Research

In the previous systematic review,[8] the team of investigators described the evidence on the effectiveness and safety of advanced wound dressings, systemic antibiotics, and venous surgical interventions, compared either with the standard of compression or with each other, in the treatment of chronic venous leg ulcers. The systematic review team noted that:

- Few randomized trials had been conducted.
- Most studies were limited by study design, study size, standard definitions, standard outcome measures, and other methodological weaknesses, rendering cross-study comparisons difficult or impossible.

- Few longitudinal observational studies of the natural history of chronic venous leg ulcers had been conducted.

As a result of the paucity of high quality studies, the systematic review concluded that there was low strength of evidence or insufficient evidence to address most components of its three Key Questions. Consequently, the review could not determine whether most of the chronic venous leg ulcer treatments studied do or do not have clinical value. In other words, the knowledge gaps in the field of chronic venous leg ulcer treatment were not merely due to a lack of studies, but to a lack of the use of study designs and research methodologies and reporting capable of producing a body of interpretable studies that produce clear results that can be compared with each other across studies and treatments. If the clinical knowledge gaps and future research needs identified in the above results section are addressed with the same types of poor quality studies published in the past, those gaps and needs will remain. Therefore, the future research needs team felt compelled to identify specific study design and methodology issues that need to be improved in future research in this field.

The future research needs team presented the stakeholders in Round 1 with 14 study design/methodology items that needed improvement. The stakeholders suggested two additional items, for a total of 16 items. Although the stakeholders were allowed to prioritize these methodology items in order for us to get an idea of what they considered the most important methodology deficits in the field, this does not mean their rankings indicate future methodology research needs, and we do not present them in a prioritized ranking here. Rather, all of these methodology items are important and mutually interdependent. Many of them are standard items of general evidence-based research widely recognized in many fields, and that have been previously codified by others.[15, 16] Other items are specific to chronic wound treatment research, and these have also been itemized by others.[17, 18, 19, 20] Therefore, the problems of low quality studies in the wound care field may be as much from lack of adherence to existing standards as from lack of standards themselves.

For the presentation below the methodology items are organized according to the PICOTS framework, with the addition of the study design and analysis categories. This is not intended to duplicate or replace existing study design and reporting recommendations such as those mentioned above. Rather it is meant to support existing standards and to highlight items particularly lacking in chronic venous leg ulcer research or specific to this field of research.

Study Design

Standards for Studying Combinations of Simultaneous Treatments

The use of simultaneous treatments is pervasive in studies of chronic venous leg ulcers, and the synergistic effect of treatments on one another cannot be determined without appropriate statistical quantitative methods. A drawback to elucidating the influence of simultaneous treatments on one another is the need for larger sample sizes for adequate statistical power. Biologic plausibility should provide the basis for testing specific combinations of treatments.

Standards for Studying Sequential Treatments

In clinical practice, patients with chronic venous leg ulcers are often treated with sequential treatments without an evidence-based rationale for the order or timing. Studies of sequential treatment strategies are especially important in understanding the best use of surgery for chronic venous leg ulcers. All patients who eventually undergo venous surgery have experienced a course of non-surgical management. Randomized allocation of participants to treatment arms is especially important in this instance because of the likelihood of selection bias in its absence. Studies to evaluate sequential therapy should have a standardized approach to the sequential treatment arm(s) in which all patients in a given arm receive the same intervention based on the same parameters (e.g., the type of surgery is based on ultrasound and failure to respond to an intervention defined in a standardized fashion). A drawback to studying sequential combinations of treatments includes the complexity of the design and the delivery of interventions.

Standards for Allocating Patients to Treatment Groups

Randomization to intervention is the best method for limiting selection bias and confounding in intervention studies. This issue is extremely important in a condition such as chronic venous leg ulcers in which the severity of disease is apparent and can thus easily influence treatment allocation in the absence of randomized, concealed allocation. Issues around selection bias are even more prominent when comparing surgical interventions to non-surgical interventions, given that surgery is typically indicated for more recalcitrant ulcers. Patients and their providers may have strong opinions about surgical versus non-surgical interventions, which can make obtaining consent for randomization difficult.

Standards for Estimating Proper Sample Sizes

Well-developed statistical methods for estimating the size of samples needed to answer research questions are readily available and should be used to design all studies of treatments for chronic venous leg ulcers.

Standards for Recruiting Patients

Ethical methods for obtaining patients' informed consent to be randomized into a treatment arm of a study—and for recording their baseline characteristics before randomization—are readily available and should be used in all randomized studies of venous ulcer treatments.

Population

Standards for Describing Participating Patients and Their Ulcers

Reporting of patient characteristics is integral to evaluating a study's external and internal validity. Knowing the characteristics of participating patients and their ulcers facilitates the generalizability of study results to different patient populations. The duration and size of an ulcer appear relevant to the effectiveness of certain dressings. Standard terms that describe wound bed appearances and a means of quantifying wound bed tissues need to be developed. Such characteristics should be described for intervention and comparison groups to determine and adjust for imbalances of confounders across treatment arms. Ultimately, describing participating patients will help to identify further relevant gaps in research among demographic and clinical groups of patients.

Standards for Defining and Classifying "Chronic Venous Leg Ulcers"

Universal definitions of common types of chronic venous leg ulcers are needed. The definitions should address physical characteristics, location, bacteriology, duration and relation to venous flow. Ideally, the definitions would be developed by consensus, promulgated, and used in all studies of the treatment of such ulcers.

Comparisons

Standards for Selecting Valid Comparison Groups

The use of an appropriate comparison group is necessary for reducing confounding and for understanding the performance of the active intervention relative to the comparison treatment. The use of appropriate comparison groups does require additional resources but is necessary to understand how study results compare with the current standard of care.

Outcome Measures

Standards for Measuring Outcomes

The valid and reliable measurement of outcomes is a major issue in studies of chronic venous leg ulcers. Most studies of chronic venous leg ulcers should employ measures that have a subjective component. As such, proper use of validated measures which show acceptable inter- and intra-rater reliability is critical to precision of observation. There is a need to develop standards for measuring healing rates as a valid intermediate outcome. For this outcome, as well as for time to complete healing, we need to agree on definitions of epithelialization and what method(s) are acceptable to demonstrate this result. Validated measures of patient-reported outcomes, such as pain and quality of life, and standards for the unbiased administration of these measures should be adopted or developed.

Standards for Selecting Important Outcomes (Primary and Secondary) and Measures

Such outcomes may include healing rates and time to complete healing, as well as safety, patient-reported and other secondary outcomes. A tool to evaluate quality of life in the venous ulcer population needs to be validated and used consistently.

Standards for Reporting Harms

All patients enrolled in studies of chronic venous ulcer treatment should be monitored actively to detect any adverse events that could be related to their treatment. All such events should be described in the articles that report the results of such studies.

Timing

Standards for Establishing the Needed Duration of Followup

Studies should be designed to follow patients long enough to ascertain the completeness and durability of ulcer healing.

Statistical Analysis

Standards for Analyzing Data

Standards for analyzing study data should include estimating power and sample size, intention-to-treat analysis, and statistical methods to account for confounding, effect modification and clustering of patients.

Standards for Analyzing Interactions Between Simultaneous Treatments

Well-developed statistical techniques should be employed to analyze potentially complex interactions between simultaneous treatments in this domain of research.

Standards for Reporting All Patients' Flow Through Studies

All patients enrolled in studies should be tracked throughout the studies, and their "flow" through the studies should be reported in journal articles. "Completers analyses" are known to be biased toward showing a benefit of the active intervention, as patients who have benefitted are more likely to complete a study. Knowledge of the reasons for losses to followup (e.g., adverse events) are useful for clinicians' and researchers' understanding of the relative effects of interventions. Analytic techniques to handle missing data are helpful and, if used appropriately, can reduce the chance of bias.

Standards for Reporting Information About Patients Lost to Followup

Studies should describe all patients enrolled and report all losses to followup. Intention-to-treat analysis and emphasis on retention of enrolled participants are essential.

Conclusions

Our purpose was to identify and prioritize the evidence gaps indicated in the Johns Hopkins University Evidence-based Practice Center systematic review of treatments for chronic venous leg ulcers.[8] The goal and scope of that review was to determine the effectiveness and safety of advanced wound dressings (Key Question 1), systemic antibiotics (Key Question 2), and surgical interventions (Key Question 3), compared with either each other or to compression systems (as the standard of care), among patients with chronic venous leg ulcers. This particular category of chronic wounds was chosen because its homogeneity would enhance the ability to make comparisons across studies. For all of the Key Questions, there were few, if any, well conducted randomized studies that provided moderate to high quality evidence. The review rated the strength of evidence of most aspects of all three Key Questions as low or insufficient. For the purposes of the future research needs reports, low or insufficient strength of evidence is the definition of an evidence gap. Therefore, for this future research needs report we divided the Key Questions into twelve individual components that constituted the evidence gaps within the scope of the review.

We presented these evidence gaps to a group of stakeholders representing clinical experts, payer decision makers, and consumer advocates. In two engagements by emailed questionnaires, these stakeholders prioritized the gaps on the basis of importance (severity and burden for patients and society) and potential impact on decision-making by patients, providers, or policy-makers.

In terms of the general categories of treatments in the three Key Questions of the systematic review, the stakeholders ranked them: (1) wound dressings, (2) venous surgery, and (3) systemic antibiotics.

Of the twelve specific evidence gaps, we chose the top nine prioritized by the stakeholders, based both on the number of stakeholders voting for a gap, as well as the fact that some stakeholder ranked it as their highest, or next highest priority. These top-tier future research needs are:

- Biological dressings containing living cells
- Collagen dressings for recalcitrant ulcers
- Dressings with enzymatic debriding agents
- Laser ablation for superficial veins with reflux
- Valvular surgery for deep veins with reflux
- Ligation for incompetent perforating veins
- Sclerotherapy for superficial veins with reflux
- Topical antibiotic- or antiseptic-impregnated dressings for clinically noninfected chronic venous leg ulcers
- Radiofrequency ablation for superficial veins with reflux

We consider our process valid for identifying and selecting these top research needs, however, we don't know that another similarly representative group of stakeholders would have chosen this particular order. Therefore, we advise the reader not to place undue emphasis on this particular order, but to consider all of these high-priority future research needs.

We searched databases for ongoing but yet unpublished trials and did not determine that any of these research needs are likely to be answered by ongoing research in the near future.

Therefore, we consider all of the listed future research needs as good prospects for those funding future research in this field, and we believe such research would substantially advance the treatment of chronic venous leg ulcers.

The stakeholders also suggested eight additional items they considered gaps, but that were outside the scope of the original systematic review. Because these items were not reviewed with comprehensive literature searches in the systematic review, we could not use the review to elaborate on the extent of these potential gaps in evidence. However, we presented a brief discussion of these additional potential evidence gaps in which the stakeholders were interested.

The lack of high quality evidence for many modes of therapy in the systematic review does not mean that those interventions do not work; rather there was not quality data to sustain such claims. The evidence gaps in this field were not merely due to a lack of studies, but to a lack of knowledge about or adherence to study designs, research methodologies, and reporting standards capable of producing a body of interpretable studies with clear results that can be compared across studies and treatments. If the future clinical research needs we identified are addressed with the same types of poor quality studies published in the past, those gaps and needs will remain. Therefore, the future research needs team identified specific study design and methodology issues that need to be improved in future research on treatments for chronic venous leg ulcers.

References

1. Raju S, Neglen P. Chronic venous insufficiency and varicose veins. N Engl J Med 2009;360:2319-27. PMID: 19474429.

2. Margolis DJ, Bilker W, Santanna J, et al. Venous leg ulcer: incidence and prevalence in the elderly. J Am Acad Dermatol. 2002;46(3):381-6. PMID: 11862173.

3. Min RJ, Khilnani NM, Golia P. Duplex ultrasound evaluation of lower extremity venous insufficiency. J Vasc Interv Radiol. 2003;14(10):1233-41. PMID: 14551269.

4. Bergan JJ, Schmid-Schonbein GW, Smith PD, et al. Chronic venous disease. N Engl J Med. 2006;355(5):488-98. PMID: 16885552.

5. Van Gent WB, Wilschut ED, Wittens C. Management of venous ulcer disease. BMJ 2010;341:c6045. PMID: 21075818.

6. Kelly T, Yang W, Chen C-S, Reynolds K, et al. Global burden of obesity in 2005 and projections to 2030. International Journal of Obesity 2008; 32:1431-7. PMID: 18607383.

7. Mensah GA, Brown DW. An overview of cardiovascular disease burden in the United States. Health Affairs, 2007;26(1):8-48. PMID: 17211012.

8. Zenilman J, Valle F, Malas M, et al. Chronic Venous Leg Ulcers: A Comparative Effectiveness Review of Treatment Modalities. Comparative Effectiveness Review No. 127. (Prepared by Johns Hopkins Evidence-based Practice Center under Contract No. 290-2007-10061-I.) AHRQ Publication No. 13(14)-EHC121-EF. Rockville, MD: Agency for Healthcare Research and Quality. October 2013. www.effectivehealthcare.ahrq.gov/reports/final.cfm.

9. Whitlock EP, Lopez SA, Chang S, et al. AHRQ Series Paper 3: Identifying, selecting, and refining topics for comparative effectiveness systematic reviews: AHRQ and the Effective Health Care Program. J Clin Epidemiol 2010;63:491-501. PMID: 19540721

10. Carey T, Sanders GD, Viswanathan M, et al. Framework for Considering Study Designs for Future Research Needs. Methods Future Research Needs Paper No. 8 (Prepared by the RTI–UNC Evidence-based Practice Center under Contract No. 290-2007-10056-I.) AHRQ Publication No. 12-EHC048-EF. Rockville, MD: Agency for Healthcare Research and Quality. March 2012. www.effectivehealthcare.ahrq.gov/reports/final.cfm.

11. DiCosmo F. The role of collagen in wound healing. Adv Skin Wound Care. 2009;22(Suppl 1):13-16.

12. Trikalinos TA, Dahabreh IJ, Lee J, et al. Methods Research on Future Research Needs: Defining an Optimal Format for Presenting Research Needs. Methods Future Research Needs Report No. 3. (Prepared by the Tufts Evidence-based Practice Center under Contract No. 290-2007-10057-I.) AHRQ Publication No. 11-EHC027-EF. Rockville, MD: Agency for Healthcare Research and Quality. June 2011. www.effectivehealthcare.ahrq.gov/reports/final.cfm.

13. O'Meara S, Cullum NA, Nelson EA. Compression for venous leg ulcers. Cochrane Database of Systematic Reviews 2009, Issue 1. Art. No.: CD000265. DOI: 10.1002/14651858.CD000265.pub2

14. Fernandez R, Griffiths R. Water for wound cleansing. Cochrane Database of Systematic Reviews 2012, Issue 2. Art. No.: CD003861. DOI: 10.1002/14651858.CD003861.pub3

15. Schulz KF, Altman DG, Moher D. CONSORT 2010 statement: updated guidelines for reporting parallel group randomized trials. Ann Intern Med. 2010;152(11):726-32. www.consort-statement.org.

16. Tinetti ME, Studenski SA. Comparative effectiveness research and patients with multiple chronic conditions. N Engl J Med. 2011;364(26):2478-81. Epub 2011 Jun 22. PMID: 21696327.

17. Sonnad SS, Goldsack J, Mohr P, et al. Effectiveness guidance document: methodological recommendations for comparative effectiveness research on the treatment of chronic wounds. Version 2.0 Final. Center for Medical Technology Policy. Baltimore. October 1, 2012. www.cmtpnet.org/wp-content/uploads/downloads/2012/10/Wound-Care-2012.pdf . Accessed October 31, 2012.

18. Schultz GS, Sibbald RG, Falanga V, et al (2003) Wound bed preparation: a systematic approach to wound management [TIME]. Wound Rep Regen 13(Suppl 4):S1–S11

19. Gottrup F, Apelqvist J, Price P; European Wound Management Association Patient Outcome Group. Outcomes in controlled and comparative studies on non-healing wounds: Recommendations to improve the quality of evidence in wound management Journal Of Wound Care 2010;19(6):237-68. PMID: 20551864

20. Enoch S, Price P. Should alternative endpoints be considered to evaluate outcomes in chronic recalcitrant wounds? World Wide Wounds, Oct 2004. www.worldwidewounds.com/2004/october/Enoch-Part2/Alternative-Enpoints-To-Healing.html. Accessed April 6th, 2011.

Abbreviations

AHRQ	Agency for Healthcare Research and Quality
EHC	Effective Health Care
EPC	Evidence-based Practice Center
FDA	Food and Drug Administration
MMP	Metalloprotease
PICOTS	Population, Intervention, Comparison, Outcome, Timing, Setting
RCT	randomized controlled trial

Appendix A. Round 1 Questionnaire

Future Research on Chronic Venous Ulcers (CVU): Feedback Round 1 (of 2)

Based on the findings of our review we put together the following three lists of research gaps in our knowledge about the treatment of chronic venous ulcers. If you feel that there are additional important gaps within the scope of the review that we did not identify, please insert them in the blank lines at the bottom of the appropriate table. Please complete and return this questionnaire **no later than Wednesday, September 5th.**

We will send you a summary of the feedback we receive from all of the stakeholders who complete this questionnaire. This will be included in a followup questionnaire, which will ask you to reconsider your initial rankings of the gaps in light of the rankings given by the others.

Gaps in Clinical Treatments

Please rank the following broad types of clinical treatments for chronic venous ulcers as to the priority with which major CVU research should be conducted (from 1 = highest priority, to 3). In deciding these priorities, please consider each treatment's potential to change practice and/or to improve clinical and patient outcomes.

	Treatment type	Rank (1-3)	Comments
1	Antibiotics		
2	Wound dressings		
3	Venous surgery		

In the course of the systematic review, we identified a large number of modalities for treating chronic venous ulcers in various clinical situations. The purpose of this section is to identify the treatments that should be given high priority in future research. Please indicate what you believe is the most important treatment to be studied for each of the eight clinical situations listed in the following table. That is, please enter in the "Intervention" column one specific intervention that should be tested first for that clinical situation. For example, in Situation 1 (antibiotics for clinically noninfected chronic venous ulcers), enter the one antibiotic that you believe should be tested first?

At the bottom of the table, please feel free to suggest other treatments that should be tested in these and other common clinical situations.

Clinical situation		Intervention to be tested first
Antibiotics	1. For clinically noninfected ulcers	
Wound dressings	2. For exudative ulcers	
	3. For dry ulcers	
	4. For recalcitrant* ulcers	
Venous surgery	5. For superficial veins with reflux	
	6. For incompetent perforating veins	
	7. For deep veins with reflux	
	8. For obstructed deep veins	
Other common treatment situations (please enter below)		

* recalcitrant ulcers are those that have persisted for more than 12 months

A-3

Gaps in Research Methods

Please rank each of the following research methods gaps as to the priority for closing the gap (high, medium or low). In ranking your priorities, please consider for each gap the following criteria:

Importance – importance of the item to the validity, consistency, and ease of interpretation and reporting of research findings.

Impact –potential to change research practices, reporting practices, clinical practices and/or clinical and patient outcomes.

In the Comments column, please add your suggestions for improving the wording of a gap description and any available information about ongoing studies that are already addressing or may soon address a gap. You may also comment about the feasibility of conducting new research that would address the gap.

	Gaps	Priority			Comments
		H	M	L	
1	Lack of standard operational definitions and classifications of "chronic venous ulcers" and "non-healing venous ulcers."				
2	Lack of a common system for classifying the dressings used to treat CVUs.				
3	Lack of standards for characterizing the patients enrolled in studies of CVU treatment.				
	Lack of standards for *designing studies* of the treatment of CVUs, i.e.:				
4	…for estimating proper sample sizes.				
5	…for selecting valid comparison groups.				
6	…for establishing the needed duration of followup.				
7	…for selecting important and valid outcome measures.				
	Lack of standards for *conducting research* on the treatment of CVUs, i.e.:				
8	…for recruiting patients.				

9	…for allocating patients to treatment groups.				
10	…for measuring outcomes.				
11	…for analyzing data.				
	Lack of standards for *reporting the results* of studies of the treatment of CVUs, i.e.:				
12	…for describing all patients' flow through studies.				
13	…for including patients who were lost to follow-up.				
14	…for reporting harms.				
	Other important research gaps that are desirable to close (please enter and rank below):				

Appendix B. Final Prioritization of Future Research Needs for Chronic Venous Ulcers

In **each** of the following three lists, please rank each of the gaps from 1 (highest priority) to 5 (fifth-highest priority) for conducting future research on patients with clinically noninfected, chronic venous ulcers.

NOTE: Use each ranking (1 to 5) only **once in each table**; do not assign any two questions the same ranking in the same table.

In assigning your FINAL priorities, please consider for each question the following criteria:

    Importance – prevalence and severity of condition, lack of or inadequacy of treatment alternatives, burden of condition to patients and the health care system.

    Impact – potential to improve clinical and patient outcomes and/or to change practice.

List 1 (of 3): Gaps in Knowledge about the General Categories of Treatments for Clinically <u>Noninfected</u> Chronic Venous Ulcers

Treatments[1]	Priority for Future Research (1 = highest; 5 = lowest)	Comments
Venous surgery		
Wound dressings		
Systemic antibiotics		

Topical antiseptics and topical antibiotics[2]	
Topical growth factors[2]	

1. The first three treatments are listed in the order of priority ranked by stakeholders in Round 1.
2. The 4th and 5th treatments were added by stakeholders in Round 1.

List 2 (of 3): Gaps in Knowledge about Specific Types of Treatments for Clinically *Noninfected* Chronic Venous Ulcers

In this table, assign ranks **only** to the five interventions with the highest priorities. Use each rank only once (do not assign the same rank to multiple topics. Do not assign ranks to the other questions, i.e., to the questions that you do not rank within your top five priorities.

Specific Interventions to be Tested[1]	Priority Rankings: 1 (highest) to 5 (fifth-highest)	Comments
Topical antibiotic- or antiseptic-impregnated dressings for clinically noninfected CVUs		
Alginate fiber dressings for exudative ulcers		
Hydrogels and hydrocolloid dressings for dry ulcers		
Collagen dressings for recalcitrant[2] ulcers		
Biological dressings containing living cells		

Wound cleansing agents						
Growth factors						
Debridement agents						
Compression garments						
Negative pressure wound therapy for edematous CVUs						
Laser sclerotherapy for superficial veins with reflux						
Ligation for incompetent perforating veins						

Valvular surgery for deep veins with reflux			
Angioplasty for obstructed deep veins			
Arterial/venous surgery for CVUs caused by mixed arterial and venous disease			
Adjuvant treatments (e.g., pentoxiphylline) for all types of CVUs			

1. All interventions were suggested, but not ranked, by stakeholders in Round 1.
2. Recalcitrant ulcers are those that have persisted for more than 6 months.

List 3 (of 3): Gaps in Methods for Conducting and Reporting Research on the Treatment of Clinically Noninfected Chronic Venous Ulcers

In this table, please choose the _FIVE_ gaps in methods that should be addressed with the highest priority in future research on patients with clinically noninfected, chronic venous ulcers. Rank each of these top five gaps from 1 (highest priority) to 5 (fifth-highest priority). Use each rank only once (do not assign the same rank to multiple topics). Do not assign ranks to the other questions, i.e., to the questions that you do not rank within your top five priorities.

Gaps[1]	Priority Rankings: 1 (highest) to 5 (fifth-highest)	Comments
Lack of common operational _definitions and system for classifying_…		
…"chronic venous ulcers" and "non		
…"chronic venous ulcers" and "non		
Lack of standards for _designing studies_ of the treatment of CVUs, i.e.…		
…for establishing the needed duration of followup.		
…for selecting valid comparison groups.		

…for selecting important outcomes (primary vs. secondary) and valid measures.	
…for estimating proper sample sizes.	
…for studying *simultaneous* combinations of treatments.	
…for studying *sequential* combinations of treatments used as wounds heal.	
Lack of standards for ***conducting studies*** of the treatment of CVUs, i.e.….	
…for allocating patients to treatment groups.	
…for recruiting patients.	
…for measuring outcomes.	
…for analyzing data.	
…for analyzing interactions between simultaneous treatments.	

Lack of standards for *reporting the results* of studies of the treatment of CVUs, i.e....				
...for describing the participating patients (and their ulcers).				
...for describing all patients' flow through studies.				
...for including patients who were lost to followup.				
...for reporting harms.				

1. Listed by category, not according to previous rankings.

Appendix C. Chronic Venous Leg Ulcer Future Research Needs Stakeholder Priority Master List

These scores have been inverted so that the highest value (5) is the highest priority.

Q#	Topic	Stakeholder 1	Stakeholder 2	Stakeholder 3	Stakeholder 4	Stakeholder 5	Stakeholder 6	Stakeholder 7	Stakeholder 8	Sum (highest value = highest priority)	Priority Rank (1 = highest priority)
	List 1. Gaps in Knowledge about the _General Categories_ of Treatments for Clinically Noninfected Chronic Venous Ulcers										
1	Wound dressings	5	5	4	5	5	5	2	5	36	1
2	Topical growth factors	2	3	3	4	3	3	3	3	24	2
3	Venous surgery	3	1	5	3	4	1	1	4	22	3
4	Topical antiseptics and topical antibiotics	1	4	2	1	2	4	4	2	20	4
5	Systemic antibiotics	4	2	1	2	1	2	5	1	18	5
	List 2. Gaps in Knowledge about _Specific Types_ of Treatments for Clinically Noninfected Chronic Venous Ulcers										
1	Biological dressings containing living cells	4	4	3	5	5		3	1	18	1
2	Compression garments	4	5	3	1			1		14	2
3	Growth factors		2	2	4	2		2	3	13	3
4	Collagen dressings for recalcitrant[2] ulcers		2		3				5	10	4

#	Treatment							
5	Wound cleansing agents	5			4			9	5
6	Debridement agents	3	3			2		8	6
7	Laser ablation for superficial veins with reflux			4		4		8	6
8	Valvular surgery for deep veins with reflux			4	3			7	7
9	Ligation for incompetent perforating veins			5	2			7	7
10	Sclerotherapy for superficial veins with reflux			4	1			5	8
11	Topical antibiotic- or antiseptic-impregnated dressings for clinically noninfected CVUs				5			5	8
12	Radio frequency ablation for superficial veins with reflux		5		5			5	8
13	Alginate fiber dressings for exudative ulcers	1		2				3	9
14	Negative pressure wound therapy for edematous CVUs	2	1					3	9
15	Arterial/venous surgery for CVUs caused by mixed arterial and venous disease			1	3	3		3	9
16	Adjuvant treatments (e.g., pentoxiphylline) for all types of CVUs			1	1	1		2	10
17	Hydrogels and hydrocolloid dressings for dry ulcers							0	11
18	Balloon angioplasty for obstructed deep veins							0	11

List 3. Gaps in _Methods for Conducting and Reporting Research_ on the Treatment of Clinically Noninfected Chronic Venous Ulcers

#								
1	Conducting…for measuring outcomes.	5	1	4	5	2		17	1

#	Item										
2	Design…for studying *simultaneous* combinations of treatments.	4	4		3	3	5			15	2
3	Design…for selecting important outcomes (primary vs. secondary) and valid measures.		5	1	2			5		13	3
4	Conducting…for analyzing data.			5	4					13	3
5	Design…for studying *sequential* combinations of treatments used as wounds heal.	3	3			2	4			9	4
6	Reporting…for describing the participating patients (and their ulcers).			3			3			9	4
7	Conducting…for analyzing interactions between simultaneous treatments.					4	1	1		6	5
8	Conducting…for allocating patients to treatment groups.					5				5	6
9	Reporting…for including patients who were lost to followup.	1						4		5	6
10	Design…for selecting valid comparison groups.		1		1	1	2			5	6
11	Design…for establishing the needed duration of followup.							3		3	
12	Reporting…for describing all patients' flow through studies.	2								2	
13	Design…for estimating proper sample sizes.									0	
14	Conducting…for recruiting patients.									0	
15	Reporting…for reporting harms.									0	

16	Definitions… "chronic venous ulcers"								0	

Appendix D. Search Strategies for Ongoing Studies

Resource URL	Search Parameters	Search Terms/Strategy
ClinicalTrials.gov clinicaltrials.gov	Advanced search, Conditions field used	Chronic venous ulcer OR venous leg ulcer OR venous ulcer
EU Clinical Trials Register www.clinicaltrialsregister.eu	Not applicable	Chronic venous ulcer OR venous leg ulcer OR venous ulcer
NIH Reporter projectreporter.nih.gov/reporter.cfm	Projects field searched	Chronic venous ulcer OR venous leg ulcer OR venous ulcer
Canadian Institutes of Health Research www.cihr-irsc.gc.ca/	Funding Decisions Data field searched	Chronic venous ulcer OR venous leg ulcer OR venous ulcer
World Health Organization International Clinical Trials Registry Platform Search Portal apps.who.int/trialsearch/	Searched Condition field, Recruitment status = ALL	Chronic venous ulcer OR venous leg ulcer OR venous ulcer

Appendix E. Ongoing/Recently Completed Studies Related to Treatment of Chronic Venous Leg Ulcers

Title/ Identifier(s)	Study Dates	Description	Sponsor or Principal Investigator Collaborator(s)	Source	Comments
1. Title: Pivotal Trial of Dermagraft(R) to Treat Venous Leg Ulcers (DEVO) **Identifier(s):** NCT00909870	**Start date:** June 2009 **Estimated study completion date:** August 2011 **Estimated primary completion date:** May 2011 (Final data collection date for primary outcome measure)	**Purpose:** This study randomly assigns patients with venous leg ulcers to receive standard therapy (compression) alone or compression plus Dermagraft(R). Dermagraft is a device containing live human fibroblasts grown on an absorbable Vicryl mesh. **Study design:** Allocation: Randomized Endpoint Classification: Safety/Efficacy Study Intervention Model: Parallel Assignment Masking: Open Label Primary Purpose: Treatment **Condition(s):** Venous Leg Ulcer **Intervention(s):** Device: Dermagraft(R) Device: Profore **Estimated enrollment:** 537	**Sponsor or PI and Collaborator(s):** Shire Regenerative Medicine, Inc.	ClinicalTrials.gov **Accessed at:** clinicaltrials.gov/ct2 /show/NCT0009098 7 0	Evaluates Dermagraft + profore compressions vs just profore compression

Title/ Identifier(s)	Study Dates	Description	Sponsor or Principal Investigator Collaborator(s)	Source	Comments
2. Title: Taliderm Dressing for Venous Ulcers **Identifier(s):** NCT00720239	**Start date:** February 2008 **Estimated study completion date:** August 2010 **Estimated primary completion date:** September 2009 (Final data collection date for primary outcome measure)	**Purpose:** To determine whether the TalidermR Wound Dressing, a poly-N-acetyl glucosamine (pGlcNAc) derived membrane material expedites wound healing in humans with venous stasis ulcers. **Study design:** Allocation: Randomized Endpoint Classification: Safety/Efficacy Study Intervention Model: Single Group Assignment Masking: Open Label Primary Purpose: Treatment **Condition(s):** Venous Stasis Ulcers Venous Insufficiency **Intervention(s):** Other: Taliderm wound healing dressing **Estimated enrollment:** 50	**Sponsor OR PI and Collaborator(s):** Medical University of South Carolina	ClinicalTrials.gov **Accessed at:** clinicaltrials.gov/ct2 /show/NCT0072023 9	Phase 0 study, very small groups, not powered

E-2

Title/ Identifier(s)	Study Dates	Description	Sponsor or Principal Investigator Collaborator(s)	Source	Comments
3. Title: FGF-1 for Topical Administration for the Treatment of Diabetic or Venous Stasis Ulcers **Identifier(s):** NCT00425178	**Start date:** September 2005 **Estimated study completion date:** Not given **Estimated primary completion date:** Not given	**Purpose:** Pilot Study to Evaluate the Safety and Tolerability of Human Fibroblast Growth Factor-1 (FGF-1) in Patients With Diabetic or Venous Stasis Ulcers **Study design:** Allocation: Non-Randomized Endpoint Classification: Safety/Efficacy Study Intervention Model: Single Group Assignment Masking: Open Label Primary Purpose: Treatment **Condition(s):** Chronic Wounds Diabetes Venous Stasis Ulcers **Intervention(s):** Drug: FGF-1 **Estimated enrollment:** 8	**Sponsor OR PI and Collaborator(s):** CardioVascular BioTherapeutics, Inc.	ClinicalTrials.gov **Accessed at:** clinicaltrials.gov/ct2 /show/NCT0042517 8	Early pilot study

Title/ Identifier(s)	Study Dates	Description	Sponsor or Principal Investigator Collaborator(s)	Source	Comments
4. Title: A Study to Investigate the Efficacy, Safety and Tolerability of Nexagon® as a Topical Treatment for Subjects With Venous Leg Ulcers (NOVEL2) **Identifier(s):** NCT01199588	**Start date:** May 2011 **Estimated study completion date:** March 2013 **Estimated primary completion date:** December 2012 (Final data collection date for primary outcome measure)	**Purpose:** To determine if NEXAGON plus compression bandaging is more effective that placebo plus compression bandaging. **Study design:** Allocation: Randomized Endpoint Classification: Safety/Efficacy Study Intervention Model: Parallel Assignment Masking: Double Blind (Subject, Caregiver, Investigator, Outcomes Assessor) Primary Purpose: Treatment **Condition(s):** Venous Leg Ulcers **Intervention(s):** Drug: Nexagon® Low Dose Drug: Nexagon® High Dose Drug: Nexagon® Vehicle **Estimated enrollment:** 300	**Sponsor OR PI and Collaborator(s):** CoDa Therapeutics Inc.	ClinicalTrials.gov **Accessed at:** clinicaltrials.gov/ct2 /show/NCT0119958 8	

Title/ Identifier(s)	Study Dates	Description	Sponsor or Principal Investigator Collaborator(s)	Source	Comments
5. Title: Improving wound healing in chronic ulcus cruris venosum with native fibrin enriched with endogenous thrombocytes (controlled prospective randomized study) **Identifier(s):** EudraCT Number: 2007-005612-91	**Start date:** 2008-04-30 **Estimated study completion date:** Ongoing **Estimated primary completion date:** Ongoing	**Purpose:** To evaluate the postulated improvement in wound healing with additive application of autologous fibrin enriched with autologous thrombocytes in the treatment of chronic crural venous **Study design:** Controlled prospective randomized study **Condition(s):** Ulcerated varicose veins **Intervention(s):** autologous fibrin enriched with autologous thrombocytes **Estimated enrollment:** 40	**Sponsor OR PI and Collaborator(s):** Sektion Chirurgische Forschung, Univ.Klinik f.Chirurgie	EU Clinical Trials Register **Accessed at:** www.clinicaltrialsregister.eu/ctr-search/trial/2007-005612-91/AT	Small study comparing aullogous fibrin with standard care; ranodmized not blinded; underpowered

E-5

Title/ Identifier(s)	Study Dates	Description	Sponsor or Principal Investigator Collaborator(s)	Source	Comments
6. Title: Evaluate the Impact of Drawtex in Venous Leg Ulcers **Identifier(s):** NCT01319123	**Start date:** October 2010 **Estimated study completion date:** August 2011 **Estimated primary completion date:** August 2011 (Final data collection date for primary outcome measure)	**Purpose:** To comparatively evaluate the impact of Drawtex wound dressing against wound bioburden in moderately to highly exuding venous leg ulcers. **Study design:** Allocation: Non-Randomized Endpoint Classification: Efficacy Study Intervention Model: Single Group Assignment Masking: Open Label Primary Purpose: Treatment **Condition(s):** Moderatley to Highly Exuding Venous Leg Ulcers **Intervention(s):** Device: Drawtex dressing **Estimated enrollment:** 10	**Sponsor OR PI and Collaborator(s):** Southwest Regional Wound Care Center Beier Drawtex Healthcare, (PTY). Ltd	ClinicalTrials.gov **Accessed at:** clinicaltrials.gov/ct2 /show/NCT0131912 3	Nonrandomized small dressing study

Title/ Identifier(s)	Study Dates	Description	Sponsor or Principal Investigator Collaborator(s)	Source	Comments
7. Title: Wound Fluid Protease Levels During Use of Novel Wound Dressing **Identifier(s):** NCT01567150	**Start date:** February 2012 **Estimated study completion date:** February 2013 **Estimated primary completion date:** December 2012 (Final data collection date for primary outcome measure)	**Purpose:** To characterize the way leg wounds respond to a new type of wound dressing, compared with wounds in patients who are not using the new dressing. **Study design:** Allocation: Randomized Intervention Model: Parallel Assignment Masking: Open Label Primary Purpose: Treatment **Condition(s):** Venous Stasis Ulcers **Intervention(s):** Device: Novel Dressing **Estimated enrollment:** 40	**Sponsor OR PI and Collaborator(s):** Hollister Incorporated	ClinicalTrials.gov **Accessed at:** clinicaltrials.gov/ct2 /show/NCT0156715 0	Biochemical analysis study—not specifically focused on healing

Title/Identifier(s)	Study Dates	Description	Sponsor or Principal Investigator Collaborator(s)	Source	Comments
8. Title: A study to research if foam sclerotherapy of saphenous trunks can speed up the healing of chronic venous leg ulcers **Identifier(s):** EudraCT Number: 2005-001551-38	**Start date:** 2005-09-29 **Estimated study completion date:** Ongoing **Estimated primary completion date:** Ongoing	**Purpose:** To determine the effect of foam sclerotherapy on the incompetent venous trunks and the effect of foam sclerotherapy in addition to compression therapy on ulcer healing **Study design:** Randomized controlled trial **Condition(s):** patients with insufficiency of the long and/or short saphenous vein as underlying cause of their venous leg ulcer **Intervention(s):** foam sclerotherapy of saphenous trunks **Estimated enrollment: 200**	**Sponsor OR PI and Collaborator(s):** Gloucestershire Hospitals NHS Foundation Trust	EU Clinical Trials Register **Accessed at:** www.clinicaltrialsregister.eu/ctr-search/trial/2005-001551-38/GB	

Title/ Identifier(s)	Study Dates	Description	Sponsor or Principal Investigator Collaborator(s)	Source	Comments
9. Title: A Phase II, Randomized, Prospective, Double blind, Parallel group, Multi-center Study to determine the Safety and Efficacy of GRANEXIN GEL in the Treatment of Venous Leg Ulcers **Identifier(s):** CTRI/2011/09/00 1985	**Start date:** 11-10-2011 **Estimated study completion date:** Not stated **Estimated primary completion date:** Not stated	**Purpose:** To study the Safety and Efficacy of GRANEXIN GEL plus Standard of Care in comparison to Standard of Care alone in the Treatment of Venous Leg Ulcer **Study design:** Randomized, Prospective, Double blind, Parallel group, Multi-center Study **Condition(s):** Venous Leg Ulcers **Intervention(s):** GRANEXIN GEL plus Standard of Care **Estimated enrollment: 92**	**Sponsor OR PI and Collaborator(s):** FirstString Research Inc	The World Health Organization Clinical Trials Registry **Accessed at:** apps.who.int/trialse arch/Trial.aspx?Tria lID=CTRI/2011/09/ 001985	